JUNG: REVISITED AND REFRESHED

A Statistician's View of Psychodynamics

By

K.W. Harrison

GW00707222

Published by

the COGAR FREE PRESS, 9 Coghlan Close, Fareham, PO16 7YE

Printed in Great Britain by REMOUS LIMITED

ISBN Number 978-0-9931818-0-1

Author's Note

The structure of this book is aimed at presenting an irrefutable case for reconstructed Jungian theory being within an environment that is most suitable for its accommodation. I have sought to develop an argument to this effect which is clear, explanatory, thorough, scientific and cogent. If, throughout this exercise, I sound bombastic and/or didactic, then I apologise and put it down to expediency.

However, there will be, among my readers, those who would prefer to know the essence of my argument in advance so that they can, so to speak, 'key-in' my points as they come to them. For such readers, I have fashioned a four-page *In Conclusion' section* to this work which they might like to read in advance. Alternatively, they might try the longer and more personal Epilogue. Or, of course, both sections.

I apologise to readers for my occasional, but necessary, introduction of religion into this monograph – I have mitigated it, as much as possible, by excluding religion completely from my tract – unless its introduction pertains to the Jung-Plato paradigm which I seek to present. Even then, its instruction will be as 'clinical' as I can make it.

This even applies to Mysticism which, today, distinguishes between 'religious' mysticism and 'lay' mysticism. 'Natural' religion is allowable in systems theory, but I only relate to that when it has pertinence of the kind mentioned above. This exclusion applies also to the Appendix, in which I present my pertinent personal experiences, choices, and attitudes.

Following Jung, in part, I have not completely 'edited-out' my own personal work and experience; and this is for a number of reasons. First, I believe wholeheartedly that experience – properly analysed and reported – *should* be considered as *evidence*. Second, I *was* there and I *did* do it. Third, the organized practice of Science is unique in the living world and is of special importance as a movement. Fourth, I hope to convey in some small measure a sense of *tone* to my narrative.

I have in mind such things as the thrill of discovery and the satisfaction of being one small part of a whole. This applies at all ranks and levels, but it is accentuated if one is fortunate enough to be in the 'forefront' of any part of the movement. There is *Romance* to be had in Science and very much a feeling of *Involvement*, and *Excitement*, and *Camaraderie*, and *Awe.*

Because I seek to be as *rigorous* as possible, the monograph will sometimes contain rather more pieces of text between quotation marks than is usual. This is intended to differentiate clearly between my own remarks, observations, reports, etc., and those of others, the importance of whose works (in my opinion) I indicate in a variety of ways.

It has been said that Presentation of such a publication can take as long to prepare as the development of the contents – and this has been (is being) my own experience. In fact, each major section (and not just Part Three) is open to new material and to consequential re-adjustment. To counter difficulties incurred by this, I have numbered *every* page – including the Title Page – in numerical order.

This may make the insertion of new material more difficult for me but, as the subject matter is not set in stone anyway, I hope it is of some help to the reader. For similar reasons, a conventional Index is not possible – it has proved possible to give in the Contents the page numbers of only the major sections.

To counter such obstacles, I have made (and am making) every effort to render the final section – the Bibliography – as useful as possible; and, in that respect, my inclusion of an author, and any annotation to his work, is a tribute to him or her. For example, I know from experience the difficulty of finding an excellent all-round teacher of mathematics.

It is very much a question of perspective and of style, 'horses for courses' in the vernacular. This is an additional tribute to the one implied by their inclusion. An example of what I mean is the subject of Supersymmetry. This is coming very much to the fore, as I write, any future reference to it can easily be tucked into the Bibliography.

A further bonus is really an obligation. I occasionally criticise an author for not being up to date (when it matters), so I feel obliged to practise what I preach.

As I write, it is exactly thirty years since *Jung in Modern Perspective* was first published. It contains a contribution of thirty-five pages under the striking title of *Jung and the Concept of the Other* by Renos K. Papadopoulos. The piece contains an equally arresting definition of the Jungian 'Problematic' (p. 54).

The 'problematic' is defined as 'the pivotal phenomenon of the composition and dissociability of the psyche'; and it is approached from a so-called metatheoretical perspective which (it is claimed) exposes a central problematic in the Jungian opus.

At the start, therefore, those few words present three radical issues. The first of these is the inadequacy of that particular *metatheoretical* approach. The second issue is whether the definition is a *metaphysical assertion*. And the third issue is that the definition excludes *Purpose* and *Priorities*.

My argument in this monograph disputes the adequacy of the approach – it *should* be epitheoretical, but it is not epitheoretcal enough. The second issue is acceptable, my thesis allows a 'psyche' to be non-material but not necessarily transcendental (i.e. *outside* the physical universe). And, thirdly, while deploring the absence of Purpose and Priorities, the thesis provides those missing qualities in plenty.

The pursuit of good practice and rigour ensures that the physical universe is considered as a system in its environment, and that philosophical propositions are given due respect – provided that they are founded upon consistent and coherent foundations applicable to both the physical universe *and* its environment.

Religion is included as a philosophical proposition under the same desiderata. This qualification means, in effect, that *all* the religions so far mentioned are acceptable for consideration because they can be developed by the twin factors of Rationality and Experience. Thus, they join with the twinned philosophies of Sino-Asiatic yogic tradition and with mathematical Platonism.

In this, I am following the example of John Polkinghorne who argues that if we can feel divine effects, then we should be able to work upon the nature of their supposed originator. There is, however, another problem with Jungian theory that has not been recognised as a 'problematic' but is just as important. It features equally prominently in the minds (and actions) of Jungians, and it has a history. I refer to the question of *Personality and its site*; and I suggest that the 'problematic' and this 'problem' are inter-linked.

This monograph concentrates upon Personality and its neurophysiological basis. It wreaks a change in Jungian theory that lifts it out of the 'quick-sands of exclusive and mutually hostile sects' of dynamic psychotherapy (pictured by Anthony Stevens) to such a level that it makes a contribution to philosophy on a par with those of Plato and Whitehead.

The significance of this can be judged by Jung's statement in *Memories, Dreams, Reflections* that his life had been 'permeated and held together by one idea and one goal:

namely...the personality'. He declares that *everything* can be explained from this central point, and that all his works relate to this one theme (p, 197).

In addition to relocating Personality into the brain, the monograph takes a step towards the kind of 'new paradigm' desired by Anthony Stevens for harmonizing the efforts of the rival sects. At present, this putative paradigm is being adopted by the new breed of 'evolutionary psychologists', and the message from my thesis is that the involvement of Jungian theory requires *categorical* acceptance of a corrected and reduced Jungian 'psyche' along the lines I indicate.

Figuratively speaking, the re-location of the Personality to the material world transfers one from enjoying the baroque splendours of transcendence, pictured originally by Jung, to grim unremitting decision making in the everyday, mundane world about us with its ceaseless succession of judgments (pictured by Jung as determining the fate of our souls).

In the foregoing paragraph, I was using the kind of adjectives employed by the likes of John Polkinghorne, J.B. Priestley and other notables, following the history of Jungian theory over the last fifty years or so. J.B. Priestley chronicles this period extremely well in his book, *Man and Time*.

He includes works by eminent Jungians in relation to underlying mathematical theory, mysticism and ESP, and to his own personal experience (which is shared by many). Rudy Rucker provides a more theoretical coverage in *his* book, *THE FOURTH DIMENSION and how to get there*. The common denominator is the work by P.D. Ouspensky, mathematician and mystic.

A subsidiary purpose for this monograph is to place into the public domain knowledge that is highly specialized and uniquely personal. The argument is not a 'hard sell' – I do not like proselytism. Neither do I like didacticism, so I beg my readers to be tolerant if my text *seems* didactic – I am trying to balance clarity, lucidity, brevity, etc., in the most comprehensible way.

This is made even more difficult by my secondary aim, which is to present Science and its underlying philosophical foundations – through computer 'models' – to the ordinary 'man/woman in the street'. I can do so only by focussing upon one particular psychological theory, namely Jungian theory, in relation to a number of philosophical perspectives. I *do* however, seek rigour.

Part One, therefore, outlines those features of subjective probability, general systems theory, particle physics, computer science, and mathematics, which help one to establish rigour, per se, and also by bridging the gaps between them. Part Two then concentrates upon reconstructing the original Jungian *opus* in respect of a modern real-time computer system and its attributes, functions and processes.

Part Three is different – it sets up what might be called, for want of a better term, an 'ideological web', which has many potential uses. The notion started off as a plain and simple Glossary, but it soon became obvious that the inter-relationships obtaining in the Glossary had important ramifications outside it. In short, Part Three subsumes and expands Parts One and Two. This is particularly clear in view of the ever-increasing powers of computers and computer networks.

Not only this, but in extension it could be used as an analytical tool with, so to speak, potential *rubrics* changing or disappearing as fresh information is gathered in. Over time, the rubrics would become more consolidated (according to the features discussed in Part One) and so a really useful inter-disciplinary document and practical tool might be obtainable.

It is conceivable that, ultimately, some kind of *vade mecum* could be developed and arranged, possibly, in terms of Orders and Degrees (as with differential equations) or 'parochial' subsets. However, it is far too early even to attempt such an ambition, and I can only limit my efforts to bringing clarity and precision to my selected Target – the problems in Jungian theory.

My hope, apart from this, is merely to plant a few methodological seeds for scientists and philosophers of the future over such complex issues. In all these respects, this Preface seems the proper place to illustrate the apparently hierarchical nested structure of Reality within which I put forward the 'refreshment' of Jungian theory. Figure 1 is intended to be only a loosely constructed outline, but, whatever the nomenclature applied to a level, some form of evidence can be produced for its existence.

[Atoms and Molecules]	The material realm
[Bosons and Fermions]	The astral planes
[Quarks and Leptons]	The causal plane
[Soul Body]	The quantum vacuum
[Soul Body]	Laszlo's fifth field
[*Spirit Body*]	
LIFE FORCE	The Infinite Orders
(YIN >-< YANG)	The Transfinite Orders

Figure 1: Realms along an Axis of Scale seen from differing Perspectives

Comment.

Walter Mons and Hiroshi Motoyama provide theoretical definitions of the entities and levels, each from his own perspective; and I hope that this figure is sufficient to show how a detailed discussion of one psychodynamic 'sect' can mushroom-out, so to speak, into an epitheoretical 'web' of significance and important potentiality.

ACKNOWLEDGEMENTS

I owe much to a number of scientists and administrators in the MoD who understood my temperament and capabilities so well that they indulged my marked preferences for working alone and for conducting original research. They had the wit and the moral courage to perceive my needs and the forbearance to allow me the maximum amount of freedom that circumstances permitted.

I received, also, a phenomenal amount of coaching – both formal and informal – which I tried to repay when executing work as a representative of the MoD or of individual establishments within it. Sometimes my sponsors put their own positions and careers at risk (see Appendix).

In retirement, I have received help from the late J.B. Priestley, the late William Thorpe, and the late Donald MacKay. J.B. Priestley gave me permission to publish extracts from his 'Man and Time' and advised me about publishers and their 'little ways'. He also solicited a copy of my putative book. William Thorpe gave me helpful ideas from his own works, and assured me of the importance of process philosophy in relation to my own work.

Donald MacKay shared with me an intimacy with ship-borne, real-time information-processing and communication systems. We had very much in common having worked (at different times) upon the same type of military computer systems. In our minds' eyes we saw exactly the same system – but from different perspectives. In fact, the two perspectives complemented each other – his viewpoint was that of neurophysiology and mine was from psychological features visible in the brain's neural networks of the mind.

The only difference between our understandings of these computer systems lay in the design principle that lies in what might be called 'an ideal form.' He believed that no representation was necessary outside the 'mind of God' and I believed that, even so, an 'image' would be necessary in the world of Plato's ideal forms.

I am indebted to Dr. Coline Covington, former Editor of The Journal of Analytical Society, for her gentle and sustained insistence that the papers I submitted to her should be gathered together in a monograph. I am very grateful for her revealing insights into the basal beliefs of Jungian analysts.

To Rosamunda, my psychagogue, who leads, guides, and inspires me, and whom I trust completely.

CONTENTS

LIST OF ILLUSTRATIONS

Figures

Tables

NOTE

I *had* planned to use diagrams that I had utilized previously, in order to show how diagrams, such as nested diamonds, graphs of step functions, and even *symbols*, can be related to bio-rhythms (as does William Johnston in regard of 'brainwaves'). However, rather belatedly, it dawned on me that this takes me too far outside my main theme, namely correction of the original and uncorrected Jungian opus. So, I left the title of Figure 3 in place, so that I could register the point that they are available. I have replaced the original mathematical diagrams by this textual pointer to my entry in the Bibliography under the title of SYMBOLOGY, in its widest sense.

FOREWORD AND INTRODUCTION

This monograph represents the final (and necessary) step in the establishment of the 'Jung-Plato paradigm'. In 1983, the former Jungian analyst, W.E.R. Mons, described Jung's system of thought as having 're-formulated the ideas of Plato in more modern terms' (p. 185),

However, as I write, the world of computers has become a 'universe' of computers and their applications. In other words, it has changed beyond the powers of description, and has made it imperative that Jung's update of Plato should itself be updated.

In striking contrast to this movement, the *ambience* of Jungian theory has changed only a little. Mons writes in terms of computer allusions to concepts in psychology, in Hinduism, in 'Teilhardianism', in Spiritualism, and so on, but his field of discourse is incomplete and shallow. However, he devotes a whole chapter (15 pages) to 'The Brain, Creator of the Mind', and another whole chapter (also 15 pages) to 'Dimensions of the Mind'.

It is appropriate that my 'refreshing' of Jungian takes place in precisely these areas. To put it baldly and briefly, I show how the so-called 'encephalization' of the Mind, and its Ego-identity', comes about through the ascription of 'Personality' (as described by Jung) to both material real-time computer systems and to the evolved Brain alike.

This obviates the single, and in my opinion vital, flaw in the argument presented by Walter Mons, namely that thoughts can *generate* 'one *particle* of mind' capable of existing after death of the organism (p. 230). [My italics] This concept clearly resembles Jung's notion of 'split-off psychic complexes', but the evolutionary brain/mind(Ego) is merely an intelligent support system discontinuous in function from its User system.

In particular, this flaw can be amended by an elementary correction to Jung's twinned pairing of the four functions of Judgment and Perception. I will show that, instead of the pairings of sensation-feeling and intuition-thinking, the pairings of sensation-thinking and intuition-feeling are far more propitious.

Indeed, they are specifics within a general movement towards evolutionary psychology which reduces the *Command* aspects of the hypothesized *psyche* to those perceived by the Classical Greeks. Namely (and loosely) these are 'Leadership' and 'the Determination of Policy' It fits admirably, too, with mathematical Platonism, and with 'ordinary' Platonism, and with the perception of the whole entity as one 'organism' being the mechanistic embodiment of an Ideal Form.

It comes about, therefore, that the overall tenor of this monograph is twofold. First, that when stripped of its alchemy, and its 'imaginative' numerology, and its 'mystical balderdash', the Jung opus sets Jung on a par with Plato. Second, that after an appropriate correction (i.e. a wider distribution of Personality) the thoughts of Plato and of Jung can be melded together sufficiently well to formulate a new, extremely powerful, paradigm.

A Jung-Plato paradigm explains, simplifies, and unites the disparate factions in Philosophy, Psychology, and Sociology, affecting and influencing everything it touches and enabling computer analysis of people and situations.   Moreover, it furnishes scores of technological models and original techniques of analysis that have already been tested experimentally, with statistically significant results.

If I had to describe Jung's ideology in a single word, then the term 'transmogrification' would be a strong contender for selection.   The natural language dictionary (Chambers, 12th Edition) gives the definition: Transmogrify: 'to transform or transmute, esp bizarrely'. I can (and will) justify both the word and my use of it. Jung's ideology – particularly as it is represented in *Memories, Dreams, Reflections* – transmogrifies the works of Freud and of Plato, and also the Hindu yogic tradition and, more widely, the 'Sino-Asiatic' tradition of today.

First and foremost, Jung erred in founding his whole effort on *Personality*. The error is twofold. He locates his definition of Personality at the wrong level and his definition is incomplete. In the former instance, Personality should be recognized in the structure and functioning of the evolved human brain – hence the concept of an evolutionary '*brain/mind(Ego)*'.

In the second case, the definition does not include Emotion (which is coupled to Heuristic Learning) and other qualities such as personal love and relationships. This is glaringly obvious today, when scientists claim that Existence is nothing but 'Relationships and Fields', and one of the greatest neurophysiologists asserts that Nature's Aim is for us to Love wherever love can be felt (see Sherrington).

This is accentuated by the fact that Jung had knowledge available to him which he seems to have either neglected or ignored. I refer to the '*natural Quaternion*', which is formed of four elements (Relationships) of which one is clearly different from the others. Namely, this is the set: Parent, Offspring, Sibling, Other.

This accentuation is reinforced by the acceptance by modern Jungians that 'the Other' is part of their 'problematic'.   This seems to be part and parcel of the apparent determination of Jung and his followers to 'see things their way'. Their philosophical stance of 'Individualism' cannot possibly be held against the flood tide of 'Relationism' - especially against the evidence I produce of the practicality of Jung's modes of Judgment and Perception in widely differing fields.

The errors creep into normative and deontic fields. It almost beggars belief that a psychiatrist, professing to hold Christian values and to be a 'doctor of the soul', should abjure all traditional modes of behaviour when making ethical judgments and to rely completely on personal ethical judgment (presumably from one's own experience and observations).

Despite this package of justified criticism (and I haven't mentioned Archetypes and Myths) I assert that, once Jung's ideology has been 'deconstructed' and 'reconstructed', it is worthy of being joined with Plato's scheme of things to form a new and powerful (and very practicable) paradigm. Plato provides the necessary goals and values, and Jung gives us an excellent idea of what Plato's embodied psyche has as its environment.

In Parts One and Two of this monograph I fuse my own research with that, in particular, of the late Donald MacKay. We worked (at different times) upon the same real-time computer system, and his physiological approach to 'mechanistic embodiment' is matched with my own psychological approach.

In Part Three, I offer an 'n-dimensional' matrix or 'grid' which serves several purposes. First, it provides a Glossary for the contents of Parts One and Two. Second, it furnishes a kind of 'road map' of the philosophical ground covered in general by Science in the modern world. Equally, it can be used by anyone with sufficient interest, because none of the categories and interconnections is fixed rigidly.

An interested layman, for example, could either use mine as a starting point or start from scratch on the construction of his/her own body of findings. In either case, their individual creations would provide a fertile ground for cross-comparisons with others. In principle, this could be done to good effect on a computer network (provided that international agreement could be reached).

However, I see Part Three as rather more than this: to me it opens a door through which our (human) thoughts can 'Mushroom' out from (or through) the Planck limits of Space and of Time into the Environment of the physical universe – we have sufficient evidence to believe this possible.

In fact, the thought comes to mind that a 'Mosaic' of notions can be formed for each 'Realm' in the *dimension of Scale* along an Axis of Scale. It may even be conjectured that Donald Mackay's idea of Comprehensive Reality takes the form of hierarchical 'nesting' of such mosaics. This leads to concepts of multiple universes (or the 'Multiverse').

More important, however, it brings us to the fact that such nesting is consonant with the Hindu yogic tradition, in particular, and, more generally, towards the mystical merging of the 'road of the East 'with the 'road of the West'. More specifically, the 'Sino-Asiatic' model is reached.

A prime example is that of a *process* as it was envisaged, say, by A,N, Whitehead. The notion of a so-called process image being implemented in or by a computer system is really very similar to the writing or enactment of a 'story' as this concept is often portrayed.

Very sinister analogies can follow, however, because the originator of the process image (the User or his/her chief engineer) may decide that the process has done its job and is no longer needed, or that it is not up to the job and is worthless, whereupon the process-image would be scrapped. The question arises, then, if the termination is not properly executed and the implemented process is cut-off from its higher realms? There are countless stories and fables about Flying Dutchmen. Wandering Jews, and so on, to promote interest.

Until now, the followers of Jung have based their various practices upon the metaphysical assertion that the characteristics of Personality relate to a "mind" and an "ego" that are part of a "psyche" which is non-material but, nevertheless, real. However, this is about to change because the monograph shows, beyond reasonable doubt, that all the attributes and functions of Personality, assigned by Jung to the conjectured non-material psyche, are actually attributable to a real-time, military computer system

It follows that, as _all_ such Jungian constructs (plus others) can be identified in such a way, then a more cogent assignment of Personality is to a "mind" and "Ego" that are generated by the neural circuits of the brain. This, of course, has considerable ramifications into the "composition and dissociability of the psyche", which is already nominated by Jungians, themselves, as the Jungian "problematic" (Papadopoulos and Saayman, pp. 54-88).

All the "personality" constructs are construable into a warship analogy that is supported by the works of authorities such as the illustrious C.S. Sherrington. He describes the human being's environment as appearing akin to "a battlefield almost from end to end' (p. 293). The construal includes such things as Introversion, Extraversion, the balance between them, Sensation, Intuition, Feeling, Thinking, the Shadow, the Persona, the Anima, Defence Mechanisms, Parapraxes, the Collective Unconscious, Archetypes, Protocols, and a host of ancillary concepts.

With such a depletion of mechanisms and concepts, the Jungian psyche still remains viable as a a greatly reduced non-material system. This is primarily because the real-time computer system of a warship is analogous to a "brain/mind(Ego) as a _support system_. The background of Particle Physics and Mathematics is an accompanying factor.

Although it was not designed as such, the military computer system follows the same bifid Command input as does the human brain, i.e. the 'brain/mind(Ego)'. The 'principle of convergence', identified by Sherrington, ensures that both systems – human and machine – employ two methods of input. One is for _normal_ conversational mode, the other is for emergency input in active operational modes involving conflict.

In the latter form of emergency input, the normal layers of input checking are waived. All the Command element has to do is to give the Command fiat, i.e. 'Make It So' or' Abort'. Equivalent processes have been denoted in the brain's neural network by Popper and Eccles.

They assert that a non-material Command element _does_ exist, and that this functionary is in every way akin to the notion of a _psyche_, held by Plato and by Aristotle, that the psyche is the _pilot_ of the mechanistic 'vessel'. The remnants of Jung's concept of the psyche show close resemblance to this kind of Command element in whichever meaning of the word 'pilot' is used.

The term 'pilot' in Plato's day was more likely to mean 'a leader into dark and dangerous places' than 'a navigator into a final port or harbour'. And the warship analogy suggests a difference between the two functions of Command and of Navigation,

Special Warfare, and so on that could emerge from 'specializations' in the neural networks.

The proposed union of improved Jungian theory with Platonism introduces another perspective into considerations. This fresh perspective is obtained from the late Donald MacKay, whose scheme of 'Comprehensive Reality' employs 'mechanist embodiment' of a person in the same way that a real-time computer system embodies a program. In other words, a person is embodied as a mathematical formula. This, of course, fits extremely well into the proposed paradigm

Working on the same 'Intelligent Support System' (but at different times) my contribution to Artificial Intelligence (and associated disciplines) augments that of Donald MacKay. We saw eye-to-eye over the structure and functions of such systems, but we differed (slightly) over the religious implications.

And so, the Jung-Plato paradigm becomes something like the following: (loosely) the autonomous self-correcting enactment of an ideal form of Relationship. Under mathematical Platonism, the 'wave-front of activation' subsumes, to an unknown extent, the functions of Command and of Navigation, etc., to produce what MacKay nominated as a 'Determinator'. [or, perhaps 'Director'?]

PART ONE: FUNDAMENTAL CONCEPTS IN ANALYSIS AND SYNTHESIS

Historical Background

To do justice to my subject (and to readers) I must devote a few paragraphs to my past involvement in it. In this respect, I started my working life as an applied statistician in the Royal Naval Scientific Service (RNSS) at the Royal Naval Physiological Laboratory (RNPL) working on conditioned responses in rats (addressing medical problems).

I ended it exactly forty years later, to the day, having prepared (on request) an outline report on a computer system (program) that could analyse its User and amend itself to compensate for his/her idiosyncrasies [This was at the Admiralty Surface Weapons Establishment (ASWE)].

An applied statistician working within a very large organization may well have a rich and varied workload. In my case, for example, I was led deeply into the foundations of Personal Construct Theory and Semiotics.   And, on another 'case', I was forced – to be able to do my job – to investigate the deepest roots of operating system design. This was at the level in which the *potential* of a program becomes changed into real interacting hardware.

The two areas mentioned above are inter-connected. They both have to do with the meanings of words (natural language words) being given numerical weights, the values of which depend upon the *context* and the particular *theme* being investigated. The importance of this being that theoretical propositions – as in philosophy - can be awarded cumulative scores as numerical *weights of evidence.*

In general, scientists (quite properly) avoid using the term 'important', but some things are immediately obvious as important. Such a case was when I transformed the Logistic growth function in Statistics into 'log(odds)' and thereby improved radar probability theory considerably.

Realising the transformation's power, I spent three days in the ASWE library searching through every appropriate book to find whether anyone had beaten me to the discovery. And, the very last book that remained contained it. The book in question was by I.J. Good, and it was entitled *Probability and the Weighing of Evidence.*

That work, I found out later, was hailed by L.J. Savage as 'a landmark in statistical history, and I subsequently published a number of papers in *The Journal of Naval Science* indicating the immense power of my transformation of the Logistic function. The first of those papers was entitled, *A Use for Plausibility in Radar Probability Theory.*

This, and much more, is covered in this Part or Chapter of the monograph. The point I wish to make here is that while approaching retirement (and afterwards) I found myself under pressure to produce a book. For example, one former friend and colleague, risen to high places, offered to provide an Introduction for it, and J.B. Priestley, no less, had already asked for a copy should my doctoral thesis go into publication.

The Editor (at the time) of the *Journal of Analytical Psychology* (JAP) was repeatedly rejecting my papers saying that they should be in a monograph. She was accompanied by the Editor of the *Journal of Naval Science* (JNS) who had already published half-a-dozen well-received papers of mine, and he wanted 'copy' from me to fill his Journal.

I, therefore, cobbled together a dozen or so ideas (from those papers largely) and he published them monthly. The response to the series of publications was staggering. Even religious fanatics wrote to me over *one passing reference* to religion. Again, pressure rose for me to publish them as a book. I, consequently, offered them to an Editor of the Oxford University Press, who was most kind and helpful.

He sent me the reviews of my offer given him by two academic referees (with the names cut off, obviously). One perceived the offering as exactly what it was – a series of disjointed pieces cobbled together – with no potential for a book. The other referee was more encouraging.

He (or she) remarked that if only I could find something upon which I could hang all my bits and pieces, then there would be something that might well merit publication. That something is the subject-matter of this book.

Subjective Probability

The measure 'Plausibility' was aimed by I.J. (Jack) Good in respect of short term *utility* for actions planned for the near future. The example he gives is that of wanting to know whether or not he would need to take with him an umbrella on a shopping trip he was about to make. Instead of considering the 'probability' of an event he considered its 'likelihood'. The same measure, 'log(odds)', was derived by me to make simpler and more accurate the likelihood of a radar 'target' being detected.

Practicality is common to both perspectives, and it is geared to Purpose. As the Logistic function is a common growth function it can be expected to represent *growth* of different kinds in different circumstances. A number of my papers in the the *Journal of Naval* Science (JNS) reflect that this expectation obtains as predicted.

More important than this, however, is the fact that the evaluation of likelihood is applicable to *propositions in natural language*. For example, Good's proposition is that 'it will rain in the next few hours', and it is easy to see how words, as signs, can be given numerical 'weightings' in that respect. 'Black' or 'Dark' clouds, for instance, carry more 'weight' for the proposition' it is going to rain' than do 'Pale' or 'Light' clouds. And, as Good indicated, such evidence is accumulative. I have used features of this kind in psycholinguistics, and I have shown that analysis can even be conducted by machine, with or without a person's cooperation.

The implications of this are substantial and the range of possible applications is 'open-ended'. However, more directly, it is clear that 'propositions' can take numerous forms, such as Ludwig von Bertalanffy's assertion (proposition) that if two processes, occurring in widely different fields, can be represented by the same diagram they are of the same type. This is called 'Isomorphism'

Isomorphism

General

The central idea of *Isomorphism* is that: 'if two systems – separated and distinct from each other - anywhere across disciplines can be represented by the same diagram, then they are isomorphic'.   One does not have to be a sceptic to see in this statement a need for qualifying clauses. This is not a problem *per se* because it (the need) happens all the time in mathematics and natural language.

The dependence of natural language upon *context* is very clearly explained by Elizabeth Bates in her book, *Language and Context* – especially in the first score of pages. And, when we are dealing with *propositions* in natural language this need is accentuated particularly because *Correct Categorization* is all important in Psychology and Psychiatry.

For example, I showed in an experiment that wrong categorization in the theory of *personal constructs* can lead to wrong treatments.   This illustration was part of a psycholinguistic experiment to replicate information processing at the 'Reptilian' level, and my report on its successful conclusion included results (factors) that were so statistically significant that I asked a colleague to check my Analysis of Variance.

However, I did not have time before my retirement to publish the report as a paper in JNS, and, so far as I know, its recommendations were never followed up – that is the 'downside' of being an applied statistician. The title of this report, 'Automation and Sex differences in Situation Appraisal', may be of interest to readers. There is satisfaction for me in the knowledge that this particular paper has aroused considerable interest at sixth form and sophomore level.

Proponents of Isomorphism, particularly Ludwig von Bertalanffy and Richard Mattessich, do not seem to appreciate that it cannot apply across *dimensions* as they present it. A few moments with a pen and paper will verify this. For example, a circle in a two-dimensional world can subtend an infinity of shapes and volumes in the third dimension, and there are numerous examples of this.

In particular, Rudy Rucker, in *Infinity and the Mind*, remarks that space-time should be supplemented by an additional dimension of *scale* (pp.31-2) – his italics.   He asserts also that Logic and Set Theory are the tools for an 'exact metaphysics' (p. x).   I take 'exact' to mean something like 'within bounds and under conditions stated'.

I say this because even with mathematical Platonism, where everything is set for ever, entities (formulae) can still be bounded, and patterns are repeated, apparently, through Realms of 'nested infinitesimals' (p. 90). This can be interpreted as particles being 'singularities of varying transfinite order'. All of this pertains to the vast concept of Donald MacKay's 'mechanistic embodiment'.

Considerations of Scale pertain also to the similarly vast notion of the strong dualistic hypothesis presented by Popper and Eccles – presented in *The Self and Its Brain*. In other words, we are still talking (loosely) about 'psycho-physical interactionism'; and

Rucker suggests that the concept aired by C.S. Peirce of 'human mind acting upon Cantor's aether-objects' might be of some merit.

There are factors to be found today that _do_ indicate that aether-objects actually operate upon the mind. But, this depends upon the definition of 'mind' as 'the software of the brain' – which is a good analogy. The term 'brain/mind(Ego)' is being found increasingly to represent the attributes and functions of neural networks and of real-time computer systems.

Karl Popper gives a discussion on 'upwards and downwards causation' in 'his' section of *The Self and Its Mind*, and Donald MacKay's focus is upon 'the mechanization of mind-like processes'. And so, in just a few sentences we can descend into some deep profundities of Philosophy, and be reminded strongly of the need for qualifiers of statements of propositions.

There are in this short excursion into philosophical foundations of meaning many 'side-branches' that I have ignored. For example, the mention of C.S. Pierce takes us into Semiotics and Linguistic Analysis treating words as weighted signs. However, I hope there is sufficient to illustrate my attempt in Part Three of this monograph to describe some of the 'nodes' in the network of 'meaning' – or perhaps something else - that underlies human thoughts and actions.

Specific

The whole of Part Two is devoted to the isomorphism between a human system of *'information processing and communication'* and a parallel system performing the same function by real-time computers and their accessories. This is where the assessment of the degree of closeness between the two systems – neural network and computer network – is important, and the numerical measures of Likelihood and Weight of Evidence are significant and much appreciated.

However, the 'closeness of fit' in the assessment hardly needs to be quantized. Reference to a hierarchical Taxonomy of System Types places the neural system and the computer system side-by-side at a very deep level. Which is fair and just, between we cannot yet define completely the differences between 'living' and 'non-living', and for many people (and systems) the category of 'hybrid' would be appropriate.

Apart from the inclusion of prosthetics into the categorization processes, the term 'hybrid' is applicable to an increasing number of man-machine co-operation in which man's powers are boosted and extended by computer systems having greater capabilities in particular areas, such as speed and size.

The areas of cybernetics and praxeology have progressed a great deal since the courageous Roger Delgrado stood with a bull in the bull-ring and used a remote control device or wand to preserve his safety! [I have the video, and most impressive it is] Apart from this, Popper and Eccles agree that a degree of psychophysical parallelism must obtain, and this is consonant with the Sino-Asiatic model discussed particularly by Hiroshi Motoyama.

The fields of Cybernetics and Praxeology have, today, been encompassed in part by that of Robotics, and Part Two will show how closely a robot can be designed and developed in a human mould. This does not exclude the concept of Command by a higher system, but it reduces it *almost* completely in the Jung-Plato paradigm following mathematical Platonism.

In all other systems in the Command Support category, an *interface* between *System and User* has to be posited. As happens so often, the words of C.S. Sherrington are helpful. Brain collaborates with psyche in an environment filled with predacity and resembling a battlefield far and wide. And, man's foes are Nature, Man, and Man himself.

We see, therefore, that the Warship Analogy – described in Part Two - for describing man in his environment. Man has to survive in order to pursue his goals – and this applies to all living organisms – they seek 'Togetherness (see Whitehead; Livesey). Sherrington, again, postulates that Nature's Aim is Altruism as Passion, and that man must love wherever Love can be felt. Such sentiments would be endorsed by the likes of Ethel Spector Person and Rollo May [and by countless poets since time immemorial - a sample is provided in the Appendix.

The central tenet of Isomorphism, then, is that two widely disparate systems are isomorphic if they can be represented by the same diagram, *subject to terms and conditions specified in their Ideal Forms*. In other words, they are isomorphic up to a specified degree of *approximation*.

A corollary is that *Categorization* is all important. There is, in addition, a qualification that even Plato thought his ultimate form, the Good, to be finite and definite. [hence my term 'specification' in line with the Warship Analogy]

The over-riding feature concerning Isomorphism remains that Jung's Individualism no longer holds good in a universe filled only with Relations and Fields arranged in Orders and Degrees. Categorization is part of the process of distinguishing the Good from its obverse, the Bad. This is Sherrington's notion of Man's foes including himself.

But, this we see is applicable to the entity that is a relation and not an individual. For example, Jung's archetypes of 'the mother' and 'the trickster' now apply to the twinned poles of a *Relationship'*. Entity 'M' and entity 'F' are poles of one non-material (or non-physical) individual. They are concerned about each other and their relationship.

And so, we find that the world of relationships is filled with processes that are wondrously self-regulating and self-referential. This is attuned to Platonism and to the Hindu yogic tradition and the Mysticism explained so well by William Johnston. In his words, mystical loving is because the individual sees himself in the Other.

The arrangement can be viewed in religious contexts or in non-religious contexts. Johnston writes largely from the Christian perspective, and so does Donald MacKay who sees the Good as the word of God. The basic notion of mystical 'indwelling' is common to both.

Be that as it may, these ideas eliminate the so-called Jungian 'problematic', wherein the individual has to choose between Self' or 'Other'. That 'problem no longer exists. The bipolar spiritual entity is focussed not upon 'Self' _or_ 'Other' but upon Self _and_ Other. We shall see how the Sino-Asiatic model has been used both correctly and incorrectly by Jungians – past and present.

Networks and Nodes

The network 'nodes', to which I referred earlier, seem also to have some correlation with the idea of 'connectors' . These are 'a superconnected few that possess a disproportionate share of all the links in the network' (Buchanan, p. 180). There must be, one feels, some significance in the fact that there are seemingly two kinds of network – those with connectors and those without connectors.

In a section on the brain's neural network (pp.61-72) Mark Buchanan comments that 'synchronous neural activity' (p. 70) appears to play a part in conscious functioning. Like so many, however, he relates to a presumed unitary consciousness, and this has been identified in seven or eight different places in the brain by neuro-scientists.

Danah Zohar discusses synchronous firing at a lower level of 'patterns of bosons' (somewhat like a 'ghostly hand') acting upon selected fermions, but there must be organization at an even deeper level to make the selections. From our point of view, Buchanan sums it up by saying 'for a computer network or a nervous system, or for a company of people who need to organize their efforts, this pattern of connectivity fosters rapid communication between disparate elements – computers, neurons, or employees' (p. 199).

Mark Buchanan links Plato with Immanuel Kant in their regard for, and understanding of, perfect forms lurking behind real, tangible objects and their appearences. The theory of networks and complexity, he says, shares a 'spiritual affinity' with there notions –even if it is grounded not in philosophy but in mathematics and empirical science (p. 19).

Scale

I thought originally of two other headings for this section – but ultimately went for the present one, which is more exact than the others. However, the two prior alternative headings furnish ideas about its subject-matter and also present a forum for my discussion. One alternative was, 'Beyond Mathematics', and the other was, 'The Likelihood of Inexplicable Facts'.

I rejected the alternatives because the former introduced a metaphysical assertion, and the latter was too restricted. During the selection process, I began to comprehend Rudy Rucker's comments that Plato did not _do_ Infinity and that Plato conceived of his world of ideal forms to be finite and definite (p. 3).

Rucker explains that Plato and the Greeks of his time had little time for Infinity. They perceived it in terms of disorder and confusion to the point of _chaos_. It has taken mathematicians well over two millennia to begin to understand its nature. And, of course, it was Georg Cantor, in the late eighteen-eighties, who started the ball rolling.

While making these introductory comments, Rucker reminds us that Georg Cantor *did* do Infinity and, even more did 'degrees of infinity'. And this not only unites my two alternatives but also rules them out of discussions of probabilities and plausibilities. It plants the discussion somewhere in the region of Popper's 'propensities', or something like them, and it limits discussion to within the physical universe.

A.N. Whitehead is my 'sounding board' for matters such as these, and he (being a mathematician and logician) sets the standard, so to speak, for conjectural assessments. He wrote *Science and the Modern World* (a compilation of previous lectures) well after Cantor's discovery of the Transfinite, so he is bound to have referred to Cantor's ideas, although not necessarily *per se*

Whitehead discusses finite and infinite 'hierarchies' in a chapter (lecture) devoted to Abstraction, and his criterion for the distinction between finite and infinite abstract hierarchies involves a *degree of complexity* – my italics (p. 209). Of particular interest to us, is the condition that 'every actual occasion is set within a realm of alternative inter-connected entities' (p. 196).

So, according to my 'sounding board' for conjectured mathematical entities, everything seems to be 'in order'. In fact, the whole Jung-Plato paradigm is orderly in this respect. Although conjectural themselves, the tenets of Whitehead's process philosophy are sound –even in respect of computer analogies.

The tenets to which I refer include the principle of Concrescence, which promotes a drive/pull for *'Togetherness'* and may be identified as 'God'. The hierarchies of abstraction include the phenomenon of *'connexity'* (209). The 'occasions' are 'occasions of experience', which are point-like entities which seem (to me) to have 'poles' akin to the poles of magnetism, except that one pole of an occasion is for 'mentality' and the other is for 'endurance'.

Order is maintained in the hierarchical organization of groups of occasions by principles of limitation, and at times the whole 'set-up' is uncannily similar to 'computery'. Whitehead's comments on consciousness bring illuminating references to the genius of Descartes and of William James; and one, therefore, thinks logically about the latter's comments on polytheism and plurality of consciousness governed by 'principles of limitation'

We must accept, I believe, that the physical universe does exist in an Environment, but we must temper that acceptance with conjectures about the nature of that environment. For example, hypotheses about 'soul-bodies' and 'spirit-bodies' do account (possibly) for many inexplicable phenomena, but how can any assessment of their likelihood, plausibility, credence, etc., be made? Except, that is, by reference to a reputable 'sounding board' or, if one is lucky, by experience.

Popper's kind of explanation, together with Whitehead's notions, seem to indicate that outside the physical universe many inexplicable phenomena may indeed be inexplicable in the Realm of Physicality. They may have to remain open to Intuition; and

Rudy Rucker explains such things in relation to discovering new mathematical forms. Always bearing in mind, of course, that Rucker sees human beings in terms of infinite-dimensional organisms.

I have in mind such things as Precognition (Priestley), Hypnotic Regression (Iverson), and Telepathy and Clairvoyance (LeShan, and many others), some of which I have experienced myself. I say this against a background of likelihood, and because in my experiences any alternative explanation of the event is sometimes far, far less likely than the reality of my explanation. Details of my experiences of this nature are to be found in the Appendix, but I have only included occasions wherein there proves to be a solid kernel of fact.

Hypnotic regression has a comparatively long history and contains an abundance of cases. There seems always to be a matching profusion of critics eager to do it down. Perhaps they are reacting to the 'wishful thinking' types who are willing to believe anything. According to reports, the latter type feeds eagerly (and sometimes dangerously) upon the so-called 'holographic principle'.

This subject is especially of interest because it touches upon *boundaries* and the *representation of information*. There have been claims recently that the physical universe contains nothing but information, but this is either a wrong use of words or a miscomprehension. In the former case, 'facts' may be a better term because it reduces the number of competing theories. In the second case, 'facts' may also be a preferable choice of word, because 'information' implies the existence of information processing equipment – there is, therefore, a logical contradiction.

This is not pedantry. We are encountering whole schools of philosophy which, for example, rather cavalierly use such terms as 'Idealism', and 'Realism', and 'Perspectivism', that imply whole swathes of different meanings, as do 'Individualism' and 'Relationism'. It is, therefore, of immense significance if even one claim from hypnotic regression can be substantiated as an instance of reincarnation.

Writing from memory, Geoffrey Iverson once produced a case in which an experimental subject 'went back' to memories of a particular church in York which she claimed had a vault hidden below it. It was then, as I recall, discovered to have such a vault. The 'Antis' scoffed and claimed that this was a known fact that she had read somewhere.

Of course, they were presupposing her powers of reading and the facilities open to her, but it is even more difficult to rationalize her report of a kind of stitching in a garment that had not been used for hundreds of years and existed only in ancient texts on tapestry. I cite this purely as a sample of Popper's talk of 'testability' and of Priestley's 'fortress mentality'. In the Appendix, I furnish similar examples from my own personal experience.

The original misgivings about Infinity, and distrust of it, shown by Plato and his fellow Greeks are being blown away as I write. Over a hundred years or so, and from the launch-pad provided by Cantor and by Whitehead, mathematicians, boosted by Rucker and by Penrose, have already acquired a very promising foothold into the subject.

I have just mentioned Complexity Theory, and now I introduce the subject of Chaos Theory. The two subjects are relevant for many reasons. From a practical or pragmatic viewpoint we can perceive relevance pertaining to Decision Theory (Praxeology), for example. Or, from the perspective of Information Theory, we can see how it relates to the broader picture. Alternatively, from an even more theoretical viewpoint, we can view its position along 'axis of scale.

This concept is almost a commonplace. Although mathematicians (e.g. Penrose), cosmologists (Smolin), and even philosophers (Popper), tend to project the axis in the vertical direction, I find it useful along the horizontal, so as to illustrate different aspects of Infinity and the Transfinite.

To me, the horizontal (abscissa) projection seems to convey, more readily than the other, a sense that there are different Realms, separated by boundaries, along the axis. For example, if we assume Realm One to be the physical universe, then sub-realms appear containing, respectively in order of size (scale) atoms, sub-atomic particles, sub-sub-atomic particles (?), and so on (This was the notation used by Popper in *The Self and Its Brain*).

The 'extension' into other dimensions (all within the same volume of 'normal' three-dimensional space) also seems to emerge more clearly along the axis of scale as an abscissa. Additionally, it is easier, for me, to insert a variety of markers, such as the Planck limits of Space and the Planck limits of Time along the route to the Infinite.

Furthermore, the positioning of entities (systems), such as the Hindu 'astral bodies' and 'causal bodies', or their equivalent Christian entities, such as 'spirit bodies' and 'soul-bodies' can be viewed more easily by scanning sideways rather than by scrolling down. This is almost certain to be peculiar to individual people, as is the case with tabular material and pictorial preferences.

This is *especially* the case with Roger Penrose's concept of *ethereality* which he posits to be necessary. For what it is worth, I agree with him. I do so because, if there exists outside the physical universe an 'ideal form', then to be of practical use the ideal form would have to be 'copied down' into that universe . This is because, in the world of computers, 'ideal forms' are (almost) completely sacrosanct. [There are obvious similarities to Platonism, Hinduism, and Christianity]

Polarity

We come now to a point whereat all the features I have mentioned begin to gel. They do so in a way that indicates both Jung's radical error of Individualism and Tmothy O'Neill's perspicacity in correcting the error. The correction rests upon the 'polarity' of an 'occasion of experience', and we note that Jung would not or could not make experience central to his psychology (see Mons). Also, notable, is the fact that, in our 'sounding board' of process philosophy, a single occasion cannot exist – it must have a companion (similar to magnetism). And, this changes the perspective to one of Relationism.

Additionally, the point comes to our notice that the term 'pole' is hardly appropriate for a point-like occasion of experience. An analogy used by Mattessich, for example, might be better, i.e. two 'sides' of the same coin – especially if we introduce as one of Whitehead's limiting principles the notion of 'propensity' floated by Popper.

The term 'pole' could then be used to indicate a push/pull towards Whitehead's 'Togetherness' from the two necessary occasions as one relationship. Jung tries to avoid this by positing that the push/pull is *internal* to the individual. But this is not so. Our sounding board indicates a *relationship* that is *external*.

Timothy O'Neill has righted Jung's error by matching Tolkien's characters, Tom Bombadil and Goldberry, with the freely-acting principles Yang and Yin of a spirit-body in the physical universe. (Outside the physical universe, they are contained within the spirit-body at a higher level (see Motoyama).

At this point, also, the first steps towards evolutionary psychology begin to appear. In other words, the likeness of a real-time, special-purpose, computer system is shown irrefutably to be in parallel with a human brain and with its functioning and sense of identities. Hence, my use of the term, 'brain/Mind(Ego).

Therefore, following on from Yin and Yang, we can look back along the stream of Evolution and search for the very first signs of their operations as manifestations in the physical universe. This must be conjectural, of course, and I am speaking loosely and personally.

I join with Roger Penrose in starting with protozoa. He chooses the paramecium, and I have a soft spot for chlamydonas - it seems a more colourful and interesting little creature. These tiny beings have open to them a range of different behaviours that depend upon their own state and the circumstances prevailing in their environment.

It is reasonable to suppose that their instantaneous action-alternatives are bipolar, e.g. 'fight or flight', according to their 'understanding' of the situation. Their internal states have a wider range, which includes all kinds of 'need', such as nutrition, self-preservation, sexual reproduction, asexual reproduction, encystment, and, if we believe in Whitehead, companionship (there is actually some observational evidence for this).

In this case, the earliest evolutionary 'information processing' conceivable is the distinguishing of 'Self' from 'Other', and the situation appraisal of 'Safe' and 'Dangerous'. After a successful action, the little creature 'marks its card' according to the conditions prevailing at the time as part of its 'heuristic learning program'. And, as pointed out by Livesey, *Learning* of facts goes hand in hand with the development of *Emotion*.

The introduction of Emotion at this evolutionary level does not in any way hinder the apparently increasing degree to which Existence is becoming mathematically orientated, to say the least. Nor does it support Smolin's assertion that there is *nothing outside the physical universe*. Indeed, many mathematicians are preaching the opposite.

For example, Roger Penrose posits that parts of his paramecium exhibit 'non-locality'. Rudy Rucker relates to 'n-dimensionality'. A.N. Whitehead has such things as electrons being constituted of occasions of experience. Cantor likened 'aether objects' pervading the Material universe to water in a bucket of sand. And, Motoyama posits spiritual forms doing much the same things in different Realms of the physical universe.

Therefore, returning to our protozoa – the paramecium and the chlamydomonas – there is nothing to stop us from associating relief from need as 'Good' and entrenchment of need as 'Bad' along the evolutionary stream almost (in chronological terms) from 'Day one'. And, in that assembly of need-fulfilment we find some vague, unfelt, 'pleasure' of Togetherness, and some vague, unfelt 'pain of Separation'.

As Sherrington (or Darwin, or Mendel) might have said, Dame Nature decreed that, from this level upwards, Evolution had a fair chance of succeeding. In short, she thought of the brilliant notion of *cross-fertilization*.   Still waxing metaphorically, perhaps she consulted Whitehead and decided to adopt one of his principles of limitation.

By this, I mean (coming down to earth) that, in general, cases of culturally approved incest are frowned upon by Dame Nature, and, if persevered with, produce infertility; and, again, Whitehead proves a useful sounding board. In the terminology of the Self-Other dichotomy, Nature ensures that Self always cross-breeds with Others, and yet another hole is punched into Jung's incessant Individualism.

These things end up, at the human end, as deep and complex intuitions and feelings that cannot be measured and are at times hardly felt. But can be *named* within Jung's schematic of Personality – as I will show and have already indicated elsewhere.

The Natural Quaternion

Althogh some expert psychologists and psychiatrists have rubbished Jung's notion of the modes of Judgment and Perception breaking down into the functions of Thinking, Feeling, Sensation, and Intuition, I have used the definitions of those functions, given by Ruth Munroe (pp. 547-8), to describe similar   processes in Radar Probability Theory to considerable effect. The isomorphism is very strong.

And, Nature has provided a framework in the form of a quaternion to assist a higher organism's Judgment and Perception in a similar way. It is ready-made, so to speak. I call it 'the Natural quaternion', i.e. Parent, Offspring, Sibling, Other. And, it boosts the Self-Other 'discrimination' in relationships. I have never seen this pointed out in text-books.

The social Leviathan

To discuss this fearsome beast I shall have to venture into allegory and into philosophical, mathematical, and linguistic history. All of these features are applicable to one man, Thomas Hobbes (1588-1679), whose original idea(s) was taken up and refreshed by the biologist Ludwig von Bertalanffy some three hundred years later.

I only mention Hobbes again to admire von Bertalanffy's choice of author and to point anyone wishing to learn more about him (Hobbes) to the entry in *The Oxford Dictionary of Philosophy* (Ed. Blackburn) extending over three extremely interesting and informative columns.

Another literary figure that I will use is David Lyndsay (1486-1555), from whose work 'Ane Dialog' the Christian apologist, C.S. Lewis, took his title 'That Hideous strength'. I use, now, the 'Shadow' of that hideous strength to suggest and to indicate the visible effects of the invisible social Leviathan to which von Bertalanffy refers.

To be as succinct as is possible, the social Leviathan distorts and subverts the natural order as it is set out by the natural quaternion. We are already in Jungian territory (from my use of 'quaternion') and clearly we are beholden to investigate Jung's attitude to manifestations of the social Leviathan. As might, perhaps, be expected it is rather strange.

In fact, his attitude to moral philosophy and to Evil serves as a marker for comparisons with the growth of 'the Shadow'. From *Memories, Dreams,* Visions, Jung said that we stand confronted with Evil as determinant reality, yet we know not what it is. Yet, he actually describes the symptoms (part of the Shadow) as 'the principle of evil, …naked injustice, tyranny, lies, slavery, and coercion of conscience'.

In essence, he attributes these things to the failing of the *Christian myth*, and that tells us a lot about Jung, himself. He, and others before him and after him, attributes (in my opinion) far too much power to myth, and this is an example. Aniela Jaffe, in the Introduction, comments that Jung 'explicitly declared his allegiance to Christianity' but that he differed in many respects from traditional Christianity (p. 3).

This was above all, she says, 'in his answer to the problem of evil and his conception of a God who is not entirely good or kind.' Without making any comment whatsoever about this conception, we can still trace and match comments from others in terms of the social Leviathan. This alone gives some indication of its usefulness as an allegory.

Jung endorsed this representation of his beliefs when the book was published. My edition [now falling to bits] was published in1964, and the work by C.S. Lewis was published in 1945. Ludwig von Bertalannfy came up with 'the social Leviathan' in 1967 (*Robots, Men* and *Minds*) and 1968 (*General System Theory)* and it is noteworthy that these were recommended books for university students at the time.

There is far too much in these books of good sound common sense applications of systems theory to quote. Two things, however, are (i) that the social Leviathan is first mentioned in ref. (1967, p. 51) and (ii) that two other particular citations are of significance among many.

They are:

Reality, in the modern conception, appears as a tremendous hierarchical order of organized entities, leading, in a superposition of many levels, from physical and chemical to biological and sociological systems (1968, p. 87).

Solid matter, this most obtrusive part of our experience and most trivial of the categories of naive physics, consists almost completely of holes, being a void for the greatest part, only interwoven by centres of energy which, considering their magnitude, are separated by astronomical distances (p. 239).

I have already outlined an allegoric description of the Shadow of 'that hidden strength' and Jungians will have recognised Jung's term for the symptoms of its presence. Loosely, Jung defined the 'Shadow' as a depository for things that were either too dangerous or too unwholesome to contain in the Conscious mind.

The social Leviathan is the entity that, among other things, fastens upon the contents of the Jungian shadow area and uses them deleteriously for the victim and for its own gain. C.S. Lewis captured this most brilliantly in his invented character of *Screwtape*, a junior, but aspiring, devil. And, in *That Hidden Strength*, he portrays the kind of hazy and shadowy system that appears to many as the kind of entity operating within so-called civilized societies.

Twenty-two years after C.S. Lewis's portrayal, Ludwig von Bertalanffy sketches in an outline of this beast that can't be seen but throws an unsavoury Shadow. He points out, as indeed did Jung, that traditional ethical codes contain no rules for complicated social systems that have arisen. Nobody appears to notice the natural quaternion built in by Nature.

The reason is, says von Bertalanffy, that

...never before was the individual so entangled, controlled and governed in his most private affairs by impersonal and hence often inhuman social forces. Moral exhortation to the individual and even his personal honesty are patently ineffective; the problem is to expand moral codes to the inclusion of higher social entities and, at the same time, safeguard the individual from being devoured by the social Leviathan (1967, p.51).

Ludwig von Bertalanffy wrote this in 1967 and I am writing this in 2014 – nearly fifty years later. Now, as I write, it is emerging that the social Leviathan described by von Bertalanffy is *not* a social system, per se, but a *hidden and maleficent* system that is covert and completely indifferent to its victims.

It grooms them, exploits them, swaps them, debases them, ridicules altruism, destroys probity, obliterates integrity, forbids freedom, encourages folly, praises secrecy, mocks dissenters and denies escape. It operates *within* and *below* society, and regrettably it has arrived largely through technology that is misused by all. Everybody suffers in some way from it. But hope remains.

Ludwig von Bertalanffy's description of a multi-levelled existential Existence sums up that range along the axis of scale that we know best, namely the sub-range from physical and chemical to biological and sociological. But, we – scientists and laymen alike – have to look either side of that sub-range. For example, Popper's declension of 'biological systems and their parts' steps *from* that sub-range along the axis of scale to cover the foundation processes supporting it – the Shadow's zone in Sherrington's 'battlefield'.

The *polarity* within each occasion of experience is ephemeral. It is a utilitarian concept that is lost immediately it is stated that singletons cannot exist. Once the two events feature in our mindscapes, then the 'poles' become Popper's 'propensities'. This is highly significant because they contribute to the building and shaping of the 'society' of events that give us *from below* a great variety of psychological factors leading to imagination, innovation, Whitehead's novelty, and conjecture.

They do so because in Whitehead's scheme the inbuilt tendency towards 'novelty' and the inbuilt tendency towards 'endurance' are just two sides of the same coin. The two different 'faces', if scanned, would present differing pictures, which could be, in principle, different 'action alternatives'.

An example of this is to be seen in conjectures proffered by expert researchers into states that have been called variously altered states of consciousness, expanding consciousness, a plurality of consciousness, and states of internal awareness. They were called to a conference by the need for research into *the domain of consciousness itself* (Johnston, 1976, p.23).

William Johnston makes a number of substantial references to a Dr. Elmer Green – expert on brainwaves and biofeedback. The Official Secrets Act forbids me going into much detail, but as always real advances in this field are being made in military systems. In 1976, Johnston was pointing out that possibilities were enormous (p. 35). And this could have been predicted even further back - since the days of Roger Delgado and the bull.

In the present context (re the social Leviathan) our main interest is the belief by Elmer Green that entities exist whose bodies 'are composed entirely of emotional, mental and etheric substance'. Apparently they fix upon any 'personality dross' and they can obsess their unfortunate victim with various compulsions. Green suggests that they can even disrupt the normally automatic functioning of the nervous system through the *chakras* (p. 99).

William Johnston remarks that this surprised him a little. His surprise was not caused by its contents – which are fairly orthodox in any religious tradition – but because it came from the pen or the typewriter of one of the leading neuro-psychiatrists in the US, who also worked for fifteen years as a physicist on rocket and guided missile research.

Analyzing these notions, Johnston comments that the most significant thing is that these indigenous entities do not operate upon the 'deepest point of the spirit' but upon the imagination. From our perspective, therefore, the notion gathers neatly together psychology and psychiatry the levels postulated by systems science and particle physics, yogic tradition and its factual phenomena, and practical experience and observation.

Elmer Green's opinions are open to interpretation *outside* religion. For example, Jung could easily (one feels) have understood them as some kind of 'split-off fragments of a psychic complex'. And, with computers it is not at all difficult to imagine a software routine – either hard-wired or not – being fed with wrong 'addresses' for their applications.

There will be many areas covered in Part Two where such malfunctions could occur, and we shall see that Ludwig von Bertalanffy actually produces examples of mental illness in similar systems terms. This will also be addressed in coverage of Donald MacKay's scheme of Comprehensive Realism, in which he features the physiology of mechanistic embodiment and to which I contribute psychological construals.

There is a sense, therefore, in which the kind of ideas promulgated by Elmer Green are enhanced and supported by systems theory's modern approach. Although still loosely assembled, systems theory has gathered in a 'systems methodology' to join with the systems science, systems technology and systems philosophy, nominated by Ludwig von Bertalanffy.

As William Johnston was airing his view on the importance and the potential of this kind of feedback, so the associated concepts outlined above were being *formally admitted* to Information Theory in respect of normative and deontic issues. Elmer Green's notions were not considered untoward in religious circles at that time – as Johnston points out.

Now, however, they have been given a wider-spread legitimacy by this formalization. W. Leinfellner, in 1974, advanced a form of *epitheoretical'* analysis. This includes a reconstruction of the background knowledge of social theories, and takes into account modal aspects, especially normative and deontic ones (see *Mattessich*, p. 261).

Finally, I would like to remind readers that Part Two presents a suggested new paradigm – the 'Jung-Plato' Paradigm – and that Part Three offers something completely different that is aimed at being essentially *useful* i.e. rather than *explanatory*. This part contains upwards of one hundred and fifty notes that are open to amendment or elimination so that they are useful to anyone who so desires to use it in any selected field of enquiry.

<u>Discernment</u>

All living organisms need the power of discernment – from protozoa, such as paramecium and chlamydomonas, to human beings, such as Everyman and Everywoman (the two are ontologically different – see May; Motoyama). If organisms lack this power, then they die. Clerics and mystics between them seem to have isolated the concept, but it *is* probably a fundamental, evolutionary and universal, capability.

The nature of 'death' is debatable and context-dependent. For example, Plato assured us that if an organism's behaviour did not 'come up to the mark', then reincarnation would take the psyche (soul) into the appropriate lower animal body. A few thousand years later, Jung conceived of a 'Creative Determinant' which measured us by our 'thoughts, deeds and acts' – which seems equally harsh in a different way. Perhaps, this might even be thought unjust, in comparison.

The issue of death also involves the nature of existence, the nature of being, and the more practical nature of physical dimensionality. For example, the trail of Evolution may involve the organism 'spreading out' and/ or 'reaching out into extra' dimensions (which seem likely to obtain).

Keeping our debate within the physical universe – but not denying an Environment for that universe – we can envisage certain features of Discernment. And, we can do so by courtesy of Jung's concept of a 'disciplined imagination', through which we can picture four elements of Discernment.

At the human level, all four elements have to be operational for 'successful' analysis of situations, i.e. leading to behaviour which, in Plato's terminology, can be labelled the Good. And, properly-functioning discernment is essential to the analytical process. In other words, the four elements of Faith, Facts, Fiction and Fantasy must be present and working harmoniously (consistently and coherently) together.

A number of things follow from this, and it is Jung's *appreciation* of these things (not his application) that marks him out for a new paradigm (in combination with Plato). First and foremost, the function of discernment *needed* Good's discovery and enhancement of 'plausibility' which enables natural language propositions to be given numerical weightings, and which allows 'fine-grain' analysis (see Appendix). A corollary to this is the discovery that plausibility is a transformation of the Logistic growth function and links numerical weighting formally to contexts and themes (Appendix).

The element of Faith, in discernment, does *appear* to be exactly the kind of 'rag-bag' of ideas which John Polkinghorne tried to avoid in his references to the noetic world, but in fact the appearance is spurious. The great power of Subjective Probability in the I.J. Good mode is that fragmented pieces of evidence re a proposition can be quantified and summed, and thereby integrated.

[By 'noetic' he was relating to his chosen context (Christianity) and he pointed out that in other contexts 'noetic' might be deemed as 'spiritual'.]

I feel, however, he may have clouded the issue somewhat by attempting honesty – in a way not entirely dissimilar to the efforts of Popper and Eccles. In other words, by introducing a possibility of inferring a substantive difference between terms that are only context-dependent. In short, he may have introduced into the mind-sets of his readers the notion of a disjunction between the contexts that is not real and valid.

For example, if 'spirits' exist, and (to borrow his terminology) there is good reason for this belief, then they might be expected to have noetic *qualities* but there is less good reason for tying-in those qualities with the term as it is usually defined. By doing so, he seems to make it a definitive qualifier of the terms - especially when he elsewhere accepts the possibility that some spirits may not be linked to the material.

Some degree of religious orientation must in any case be accepted because Polkinghorne *is* making a case for Christianity. However, I do not accept this as a reason for loading words without notice. A similar infelicity occurs when he says 'When all is said and done, quantum fields are simply creatures' (1988, p.58).

I point these things out not from pedantry, but rather because they are part and parcel of an attempt by John Polkinghorne to discuss the concepts of Platonism and of

Whitehead in a comparative study re Christianity. They are consequently at the very heart of my thesis. For example, in contrast to my use of Whitehead as a 'sounding board', he dismisses process philosophy as 'baroque grandeurs' (p. 83).

A smile comes to one's lips when, in the same sentence, he asserts that the physical world 'participates in a wider noetic field, *all being held in being by the creative will of God* (my italics). Now, a critical point has been reached, because the machinery *by which this takes place* (my italics) is the 'humble picture of material/mental complementarity' (my italics).

Material/mental complementarity is context-dependent – it depends upon the definition of 'mental'. And, John Polkinghorne argues that 'the mutuality of mental and material is relevant to the insights of quantum theory about the structure of the physical world' (p. 77). He describes the constituent roots of the material realm as being the cloudy and fitful realm of 'quantum unpicturability'. However, *mathematical* Platonism excludes this 'unpicturability'.

Classical Platonism differs, he says, in two important aspects from the view that he advocates. The first is that it 'in no way assigns a priority to the mental over the material'. But, this proposition is based upon the term 'mental' being applicable to what in another context might be termed 'spiritual', whereas we know today that the term 'mental' is properly assigned to the Mind(Ego) as the software of the material brain.

Thus, in those circumstances, we can still conceive of the spiritual noetic entity, to which he refers, as the 'User' of the 'brain/mind(Ego) and relate it to an overall picture of Command. But, the action, so to speak, still pertains to the realm of the material. Moreover, the 'austere abstractions of mathematics' would still be present as Plato's ideal forms.

The notion of ideal forms is boosted by isomorphism between the brain and a special-purpose real-time computer. The isomorphism is beyond doubt, and in part this is due to Donald MacKay's concept of 'mechanistic embodiment' being exemplified by a mathematical formula actually *being* the embodiment.

MacKay addressed his efforts towards 'the mechanization of mind-like processes' in terms of such a computer system, and, in Part Two, I amplify and complete his idea by providing a mechanized 'Personality' (complete with all its features characteristic of Mind and Ego) for that system. Over a chain of correspondence he agreed that we conceived of exactly the same type of system – but this is not surprising because (at different times) we had worked upon the same system.

However, this does not preclude a 'spiritual' User of the system – although we disagreed about the existence of the 'ideal form'. We saw eye-to-eye about the User being the implementation of an ideal form, but MacKay saw no need for it to be part of the Platonic world because it already was held in the 'mind of God'. Our only difference of opinion, therefore, was a matter of Faith.

All of this swings into place by replacing the cloudy and fitful world of quantum unpicturability by mathematical Platonism wherein everything is fixed (see Roger Penrose). The reality of quarks, gluons and electrons holds good. What happens is that a wave of excitation sweeps through the fixed world of mathematical Platonism, ordered and directed from outside the material universe.

For our purposes, this is sufficient – there is no need to go further, into the transcendental.   For all of these conjectures, we have not only the sounding board of Whitehead's system of thought, but also the *physical model* presented from the hard facts of real-time computer systems.

In summary, therefore, we can say the following:

Deconstructed and re-constructed Jungian theory merges neatly with Platonism to provide a paradigm that is Just and Autonomous.   Mechanistic embodiment ensures that this arrangement produces the balance sought by John Polkinghorne between the material and the spiritual.   Divine intervention is allowed under the epitheoretic scheme, which is consonant with Mysticism and Natural Theology.

The paradigm is based upon mathematical and technological foundations which furnish opportunities for modelling by computer and for testing, experimentation and validation by subjective measures of evaluation.   Its experiential orientation is consonant with not only Christianity but also Hinduism in its yogic traditional form.

Process Theology can be more useful as a 'sounding board' than as a model.   As such, it lends support to the definitions of 'soul' and of 'spirit' that emerge from evolutionary studies.   Discernment is part of the evolutionary process and it enables a (Jungian) quaternion to be envisaged in which the four elements are the functions of 'situation assessment' and the element that is different is the element of Faith.

The four elements form a structural hierarchy of 'Fantasy', 'Fiction', 'Fact' and 'Faith', and they are not mutually exclusive.   The 'highest' element is not 'blind faith' but 'reasoned faith', and it includes such things as Tertium Organum (i.e. intuitive logic) and 'Quartic Organum' (mystical insight and apperception.   It may, or may not, include Quintic Knowledge (i.e. Revelation).

Discernment is an apt word in the Jung-Plato paradigm because the 'embodied mathematical formula', with its spiritual 'elective' (or eclectic) affinity as its guide, has only to select the right path to reunion from a miscellany of alternative paths.   Its guide is its real 'soul-partner' which, in effect, is recollected and, therefore, becomes a 'soul-constant'; and the guide or 'soul-image' is necessary because there is a multitude of 'close-fits'.

A mathematician might, indeed, say that the arrangement has a beautiful balance and symmetry.   A cyberneticist would probably agree.   The relationship is self-correcting: each pole of the relationship contributes to it.   In the kind of mystical language used so well by William Johnston 'each sees itself in the Other'.   And, this is where Jung went so grievously wrong by his espousal of Individualism.

The 'entity' is a 'spirit-body' or field, and Its two 'poles' are parts of that entity manifested in lower realms as material bodies.   They can operate and co-operate because the entity exists if three-dimensional time; and we know this partly from our experiences (shown by Priestly to be more commonplace than expected) and partly because its existence has been shown as mathematically plausible by J.B. Priestley's friend, J.G. Bennett.

I opine that J.B. Priestley made a more valuable contribution to science than is expressed generally. Even his exasperation with 'closet scientists' who refuse to consider any phenomena than 'their own' is valuable not only for the 'easing in' of non-testable phenomena, but also for the identification of those with a 'fortress mentality' that impedes and injures scientific progress.

After forty years of cross disciplinary research I would dearly love to add examples, but I have been strong for a further twenty-six years and I will not give way now (despite inducements). So, I continue and point out that modern day scientists appear to be little better than they were in my day – if that in some very few instances).

Changing the subject, Lee Smolin is well regarded, and he eclares that there is nothing outside the physical universe and that the physical universe consists only of relationships and fields. In my opinion, the first declaration is debatable and the second is eminently reasonable. I am not sure about his further reduction, i.i. the statement that there is only 'Information'. To me, the presence of 'information' implies the existence of information-processing, which implies 'entities' pursuing such activities.

Discernment and its sub-functions are processes and sub-processes, and the information upon which they operate is *Evidence* which can be ordered and arranged in relations to contexts and themes. Broadly speaking, for example, we can associate categories of information with the appropriate functions and sub-functions along the evolutionary trail until new categories *emerge*.

I emphasize *emerge*, wishing to make the point that they *emerge into view*. They are discovered rather than created, and in that sense it is beginning to emerge that Existence is tiered and *real*. Rudy Rucker's words apply concerning the One and the Whole. The Hindu yogic tradition swims into focus; and so on.

In fact, it might be said that the discovery of 'plausibility' associated with 'weight of evidence' and the growth of information, opens the way to (i.e. enables) the consideration of formal and logical issues of extreme importance existing at much deeper levels of mathematical statistics. Possibilities of establishing *central order* are to be seen, and also of *confidence limits*. And, Rucker's concept of a *dimension of* scale is completely ratified.

With that ratification comes the concept of using statistical operators which are 'consistent and asymptotically normal and asymptotically efficient for large samples under general conditions'. Some estimators are open to bias, but 'frequently the bias can be removed by a simple adjustment (Brownlee, p. 91). The linkage between subjective probability and the Logistic function inevitably comes to mind, but I have not had sufficient time to pursue this further.

I will say that, speaking from experience, the amenability with which the logistic function absorbs different probability distributions over successive time intervals invites the notion that the dimension of 'Scale' contains an 'axis of scale' along which differing

'Realms' of Existence' be sectioned off   as in Hinduism's yogic tradition and 'Logistic mapping'.

For example, we already have, in particle physics and in Jungian theory, the first four such Realms (atoms, sub-atomic particles (fermions and bosons), sub-subatomic particles (quarks and leptons), and sub-sub-subatomic particles (so-called 'virtual particles').   Considering that the axis of scale is measured in terms of logarithms, it might just be more profitable to think a bit more statistically before planning vast expenditures of time and effort on experiments of the 'suck-it-and-see' type.

There are also 'second order' effects to be from using this perspective.   I refer to discoveries being made in associated disciplines such as Chaos theory and Complexity theory which are not so directly related to the logistic function.   An example of this would be the 'Mandelbrot set' which is produced by the function that appears to run along the axis of scale and to pass through all the realms.   Various other functions can be accommodated also, all of which go to show how very useful are both the logistic function and the notion of scale as a dimension.

One final commendation of mathematical Platonism is that it restores the kind of picture painted by Sherrington of the collaborative brain using a principle of convergence to support an 'ultimate (psychical) pontifical nerve-cell'.   Since Popper and Eccles published *The Self and Its Brain* Sherrington seems to have been completely forgotten. Yet, he portrayed exactly the process of Command as it exists in a warship.

In this context, Command is ephemeral – it is the *entity* as a whole that is charged with missions.   Donald MacKay, having (as do I) intimate knowledge of the support system, calls the organismic equivalent, *the agent,* and the Command's organismic equivalent, *the determinator*.   The crucially important thing is that both functions are lodged within the same embodied mathematical formula.   This fits perfectly with, and only with, Platonism.

Isomorphic Categorization

The term 'isomorphic categorization' would sound grandiloquent, and smack of jargon, in the hands of an author such as Ludwig von Bertalanffy or Richard Mattessich. All too often, however, it stems from translation from one natural language to another. Sometimes it is even unavoidable – and plenty has been written about this.

Yet, the concept is of fundamental importance, and has much potential utility and value, as the prime feature of this monograph.   The term merely relates to the formation of personal ideas in one's brain/mind and the way in which they become marshalled and packaged as personal constructs or *categorizations*.

I have already shown (see Bibliography) how errors in categorization can lead to wrong diagnosis and even erroneous treatment in clinical practise.   But, in this book, I use the term in reference to the *inter-dependence* of Science and Philosophy upon each other and their *mutual* dependence upon a welter of notions from *all* disciplines melded together as a consistent and coherent platform.

In short, I am describing – in Parts Two and Three – an *'Imperative '* for both Science and Philosophy to cross boundaries that have become entrenched within the two disciplines, so that their efforts rest upon sound foundations common to both disciplines.

These foundations may well have been far less secure without contributions from Subjective Probability, the 'logico-mathematical' thesis of General System Theory, and the mechanistic embodiment provided by Comprehensive Realism, which form the 'weft and warp' of both disciplines.

PART TWO: CHARACTERISTICS OF INTELLIGENT SUPPORT SYSTEMS

INTRODUCTION

On Things Metaphysical

In this part of the monograph I deal with information processing systems of one particular *material* type.   Before that, however, I must indicate certain features pertaining to that category of material systems..

In Part Three, I will make available two things.   First, I will furnish some of the multiplicity of 'facets' or 'aspects' (pace von Bertalanffy) of Existence from which I have formed (together with Experience, including Emotions) my personal body of beliefs on that matter.   That individual assembly of 'facets' of experience has led me to think it more likely than not that something similar to the 'Jung-Plato' paradigm obtains.

As a statistician, I cannot bring myself to proclaim anything more rigorous than this.   However much I may hope (and pray) that certain features of my experience are real effects, it may well be that they are 'all in my mind'.   There are certain inexplicable features, mentioned in the Appendix, that give me great cause for hope, but I believe (as much as I believe anything), that one is not encouraged to pray for oneself.   And so, I pray for relationships of which I form a part.

Each of the revealed religions contains a feature, or features, of which I can only say 'But That I Can't Believe', as did the former Bishop of Woolwich, Dr. John Robinson. But, I beg my readers to accept that Part Three contains very little 'wishful thinking' or even conjecture – so far as possible I identify *facts* and *relations* between facts.

I accept the plea of many scientists that they have no time to spare for the consideration of the philosophical foundations of their disciplines – in Part Three (without being vainglorious or patronizing) - I have done some of this work for them.   I cannot praise the Institute of Statisticians too highly for their attitude in such matters.   In their Final examination papers they have included papers on the philosophical foundations of Statistics, selection of staff, information flow, the treatment of error, and so on.   [this was many years ago].

Finally, I must give my own position on Religion.   It is an expanded form of Natural Theology which takes as a given that Science is bound up with metaphysics (Thorpe, p. 1). Also, that Metaphysics is (from Whitehead quoted by Thorpe) 'an endeavour to frame a coherent, logical, necessary system of general ideas in terms of which every element of our experience can be interpreted'.   [William Thorpe's citation is from Whitehead's *Process and Reality*, but a better source might be *Science and the* Modern *World* which is just as informative and easier to read].

Natural Theology is defined as 'Doctrines concerning God that are attainable by natural processes of reasoning, as opposed to those that require the assistance of revelation' (The Oxford Dictionary of Philosophy, p. 256).   And, by 'reasoning' I mean 'acquiring knowledge' in ways other than revelation.

This naturally includes Aristotle's 'Organum' of Deduction, Bacon's Organum of Inference, Ouspensky's Organum of Intuition, and the shared 'experiential knowledge' from mystical indwelling - which is within my own experience and is only feasible by such a process. [This does not imply that I reject, categorically, an Organum of Revelation]

My term 'expansion' includes the wisdom and knowledge written up by Freudian psychiatrist Ethel Spector Person and by existentialist psychiatrist and philosopher, Rollo May. The former explains in detail the various circumstances of Love as an Agent of Change, and her work is geared to medical experience and practise –and I can endorse that from experience.

Rollo May's perception of Love as an ontological necessity is a metaphysical assertion, although it stems from clinical practice also, and so I cannot endorse it although it seems eminently reasonable. However, I *do* endorse *some* of the findings of William Johnston, re neurophysiology, and of Hiroshi Motoyama, re system structure and function and computers, because I know that they are correct.

The second thing that I offer in Part Three (and not in any way of condescension) is a methodological tool which can be used by anybody to gain secure knowledge and understanding of *anything*. In this capacity, the 'node/network' approach that I have used to formulate the paradigm is based on facts.

The facts are that (i) people actually do hold opinions (but not the contents of their opinion), (ii) results from my own research (invited by the authorities) in linguistic analysis (the results of which were given extra-special statistical analysis), and so on. And, a factual part of all this includes those facts from subjective probability concerning the weighing of evidence and the nature and *value* of that evidence. These and other things are the facts of MacKay's Comprehensive Realism.

Systems Theory (or, if preferred, General System Theory) *invites* or *encourages* notions of deity and/or superordinacy, but it does *not* suggest deism or theism. It perceives hierarchy and nested forms of union or re-union but this does not lead to Aristotle's Prime Mover and certainly not a Prime Mover who 'holds everything together moment-to-moment'.

Suppose, for example, we gave an ant human powers of analysis (possible under Plato's scheme of metempsychosis) with it living in Roman times, it could perhaps be expected to perceive and to applaud the various forms of 'triumph' (including wondrous organizational powers and individual powers of discipline and self-sacrifice leading to the triumphs), but the little creature could hardly be expected to conceive of the vicissitudes suffered by all and sundry under the crazed excesses of emperors in the Roman world at its worst.

An axis of *scale* is essential for envisaging the immensitude of Existence, and the logistic function for separating out Realms along the axis. Outside the Realms of the physical universe there is not nothing (as postulated by cosmologist Lee Smolin) but *everything*, because it is almost a commonplace that, in the finest grain, everything reduces to *spirit* – both inside and outside the physical universe. And, we remember that mathematician, Rudy Rucker, suggests that Scale might be a *dimension*.

This takes me to the differences that have crept into Christian theology between the dogmatism of the organized Church and the structure and function (i.e. the mechanics) of the world in which Jesus Christ preached the Gospel. Which, for me, centres upon the words of Jesus as they have been reported by various contributors to the Bible.

It takes me, also, to the religious underpinnings of Comprensive Realism (Donald MacKay) and of Walter Mons (Jungian psychiatrist) and of the mechanics of the Hindu yogic tradition (described by Hiroshi Motoyama). And, straightaway, I must declare that the words of Motoyama not only link (overlap) with Mons and with Plato, and with Mackay, but also expand upon them to bring in 'the Cantorian contribution' and fit them into the axis of scale.

W.E.R. Mons had an estimable career in Jungian psychiatry behind him when he wrote *Beyond Mind* and his book is full of very quotable phrases and paragraphs, although it is illogical and inconsistent. It is not a bad source book, but is a very bad exemplar and not to be followed.

I say this with confidence, having looked quite deeply into *Beyond Mind*, and I can give my reasons quite succinctly. Mons pursued his Jungian inclinations too vigorously and in the wrong directions. He followed Individualism when he should have followed Relationism and advocated an impossible kind of 'dualism of substance' rather than a 'dualism of properties'. His attitude towards Christianity was, to say the least, unbalanced and tangential.

I must give an example, and it is as follows (my italics throughout). He basic notion is that Evolution aims at *perfecting* a *brain* in which *thought* can give rise to one *particle* of a *mind* which can continue to exist after the death of the organism. Those particles develop until ultimately they all reach the same state of perfection in which they lose their identity and merge into one single Spirit.

There is a great deal of Jung in this – much of which has to be written-out in view of today's concept of a physical universe in which there are only relations, fields, and interactions between them. Cyril Burt's notion of a field of force interacting with a field of information is excellent, and it can be exemplified in terms of a program consisting of holes punched into paper tape (which has many metaphysical ramifications).

Nevertheless, the ideas of Walter Mons – apart from 'transubstantiation' and 'perfection' *can* be accommodated by replacing the former term by something like 'relational holism' or 'holistic dualism' , e.g. dualism by properties (which reaches down into mathematical physics), and changing the latter into something akin to 'completion' in terms of differing levels within nested hierarchies.

Therefore, I will confine my selection of information only to those pertaining to the Jung-Plato paradigm. And, what better place to start than Sex – other than Love, of course. Mons points out that Freud was successful in showing that male sex-desire is hidden behind even the most harmless symbolism (p. 47).

He then continues to remark that Jung's aversion to Freud's theories led him to the 'other extreme of ignoring sexual implications even when they were obvious' and discounting inferences behind this because Jung, as a therapist, knew perfectly well that periodic dreams about sex are normal in a man, and that 'a certain preoccupation with sex is also normal – as long as his sex-object is normal too'.

This remark supports criticism of Jung's exclusion of personal love from his ideology and his delegation to God only of 'cosmogonic' love – this is relevant clearly to the paradigm.   But it is secondary to his (Mons's) focussing upon the list of man's constituents given by Dr. R. Crookall and the identification of the Hindu chakras – both on the same page (p. 194).

This list, and the accompanying chakras (and nadis), runs parallel to Hiroshi Motoyama's outline of the general 'Sino-Asiatic' structures and functions.   These concepts cover Existence along the whole conjecturable length of the axis of scale, of which the physical universe is only a small part.   They are vastly different from Mons's picture of the physical universe covered by an evolved spiritual shell.

Crookall's list (echoed by Motoyama) is as follows:-

- The familiar physical body
- A semi-physical vital body or vehicle of vitality by which it is animated;
- A super-physical Soul-Body using the other two bodies and animated by
- A true, transcendental Spirit-Body - formless radiation rarely perceived.

Comparing this with Mons's account, we find in Mons two salient differences. The first of these is the evolution of a spiritual soul from the brain/mind (instead of a mechanistically embodied soul).   The second is the absence of a hierarchic set of levels of divinity extending into and past the Transfinite.   There is, also, a retention of 'perfection' – a notion dispelled by Medawar long ago (this is replaced by the idea of 'completion').

The Jung-Plato paradigm is therefore supported by the Sino-Asiatic model, which has a remarkable integrating effect.   In regard of Plato, Plato's more general concepts are bonded with mathematical Platonism, and the result is joined with a structured portrayal of the Infinite and the Transfinite (the classical Greeks felt unease about Infinity – see Rucker).

Particle physics is joined with 'corrected' Jungian theory to link with Platonism as a whole and, in effect, this nullifies the bitter criticism levelled by Mons at Christian dogma, in general, and at Jesus Christ, in particular.   It does this by emphasizing that Christian precepts, other than dogma, are applicable to much the same kind of territory as is addressed by Mons.   That is to say, they are 'localized' in the ways presented to us by William James, William Johnston, et al.

In short, everything seems to be subsumed within the Sino-Asiatic system of thought. Even Mons's hostility to the 'miracles' wrought by Jesus Christ is swept away by the notions of 'Cosmic Parochialism' and 'Holistic Relationism', i.e. the reversal of Danah Zohar's 'relational holism'. (see Cosmic Parochialism; Holistic Relationism; in Part Three).

This seems an admirable point at which to start discussing what could be called 'physical isomorphism' and which includes the four realms covered by both particle physics and the Sino-Asiatic model.   This stretches from the material (atoms), through the realms of sub-atomic particles (fermions and bosons) and sub-sub-atomic particles (leptons and quarks), and down to the 'quantum vacuum'.

Things Materially Isomorphic

The 'Jung-Plato Paradigm' is founded primarily upon a deconstruction and reconstruction of Jung's ideology, which is long overdue. If I had to describe the nature of Jungian theory in a single word, it would be 'Transmogrification' (and W.E.C. Mons seems to be following suit in that process – but in a different direction).

The natural language dictionary (Chambers, 12th. Edition) defines the term: 'Transmogrify – to transform or transmute, esp bizarrely'. I can and I will justify my use of the term. Jung's ideology – particularly in *Memories, Dreams, Reflections* – transmogrifies the words of Freud and of Plato, and also the Sino-Asiatic paradigm or more specifically the Hindu yogic tradition.

First and foremost, Jung erred in founding his whole philosophy on *Personality*. The error is twofold. He locates it in the wrong Realm (in the Realm of Spirit instead of Matter), and his definition is incomplete. Personality is recognisable in the structure and functioning of the evolved human brain, i.e. the neural system.

His definition does not include Emotion (as Mons and others have pointed out). This is glaringly obvious today, when we have cosmologists claiming that the physical universe is nothing but fields and relations, and great psychotherapists informing us that 'Love is an agent of change' and is an 'ontological necessity'. Additionally, with a most eminent neurophysiologist assuring us that Nature's Aim is 'Altruism as Passion'.

The 'warship paradigm' is most appropriate and cogent in respect of Sherrington's other observation that man's environment is like a battlefield far and wide. But, for brevity, comprehensibility, cogency and rigour, it suffices for me in this part to describe in some detail just how isomorphic are the brain and the computer system, together with their underlying Purpose, which is 'survival in order to pursue purpose'.

Donald MacKay has provided for the physiological aspects of the human organism, and this Part contributes to his scheme by providing the *psychological* parallels between a material brain/mind(Ego) and a special-purpose real-time computer system. Although the contents are very largely Jungian, other commonplace psychological effects are included, such as nervous tics, defence mechanisms, processing of input, etc. There are also functions applicable to all life forms, such as 'protective mimicry' and 'predatory mimicry'.

From whole rafts of perspectives, such those as given in Part Three, it appears 'only to be expected' that Personality, Judgment, and Mind, should prove to be functions and attributes of an evolved material brain. The only thing that might be said about these attributes and functions being 'psychical', i.e. non-material, is that it does not (if it exists at all) run completely parallel to the material brain (see Popper and Eccles on Parallelism).

However, (see Kent), these 'mental' processes of *both Man and machine* are identical with those ascribed by Jung to the psyche. They lie, as Jung himself asserted, at the very heart of his psychology. After 'encephalization', however, the non-material *psyche* is left to be considered only in a role of 'navigator' or 'pilot' or 'determinator' or 'director', described by Sherrington as a *supreme, ultimate pontifical nerve-cell*.

I will, therefore, describe first Extraversion, Introversion, Thinking, Feeling, Sensation, and Intuition exactly as they obtain in the computer based, real-time 'Intelligent Support System' of a modern warship. Having done this, I will go on to furnish other Jungian features, and then, lastly, the functions common to both warship and ISS that are *not* specifically Jungian but more or less common to all psychologies.

An Intelligent Support System has Identity and Awareness, both of which are compound and hierarchical. The identity is represented by a unique number categorizing it as a particular kind of software system, together with identifiers of its specificity within the category for the benefit of self-reference and for its communications with others, e.g. in networks. [A robot would have the same].

The compound nature of Awareness is principally a matter of level. For example, one large area of interest is the management of 'own' individual processes; and, of equal importance (but 'higher' in level) is the dealing with others in the environment, not only in the present but in the past (analysis) and in the future Prospection).

In a human system the distinction is made between the two centres of awareness that span the whole evolution of the brain – from brain stem to cerebral cortex. Common to both man and machine is the division of labour between the cerebral hemispheres (no evidence has been found for this being deliberate modelling].

There is a clear distinction of function in both kinds of system (man or machine), also, because the one deals exclusively with the workings of the whole brain itself, whereas the other kind of awareness engages the attentions, outwards and forwards, of the 'feed-forwards' mechanisms of the brain.

Ernest Kent believes that this is enough for a monistic viewpoint – but he is wrong. His conjectural computer system does not allow for it being a *support* system. He mistakes part of the operating system for the so-called 'ultimate pontifical nerve-cell'. It is worthy of note that brain systems and computer systems are each built up from the simplest components, such as clocks, timers, interrups, flags, etc., etc., and that they both exhibit periodicity and cyclicity.

This gives even more power to the use of *functional models*. G. Spencer Brown emphasizes this point. He maintains that it is not enough for science to look for models of likeness alone. It looks for Functions; and a function is a working (or workable) model of a changing or changeable state of affairs. Modern systems theory copes with this adequately, and his point that to find or make up likenesses is to find or make up *relationships* (p. 13) is exactly the thrust of General System Theory.

So, even before beginning to discuss the four functions constituting *Perception* and *Judgment* in a warship's Intelligent Support System, we find in it (a) hierarchical plurality of awareness, (b) completely separate and distinct functions and roles, and (c) *Purpose* completely different from the Jungian conception.

The warship's purpose is completely 'Other-orientated', and , for the Jungian, purpose is 'Self-orientated'. Jung's words are: 'the goal of psychic development is the self'. However, this difference is eliminated with encephalization, whereby the concept of *Individuation* is virtually identical in warship and human. The aim is to make *organism* as a whole fully operational.

FEATURES TYPICAL OF ACTION SYSTEMS

(i) THE ENTITY IN ITS MILIEU

Ludwig von Bertalanffy and Richard Mattessich might well have used the term 'Isomorphism' in reference to these features, but it is probably more rigorous to be more specific – hence my title for this section. There are numerous reasons for this, but the book, *Action Systems*, is closer to my approach and mind-set.

The authors, David D. Clarke with Jill Crossland, express the hope (p. 146) that it will enable psychologists, linguists, engineers, computer scientist, and others to 'take a fresh look' at 'natural action in all its complexity, and in the full richness of the systems which it forms'. This is the underlying and unifying theme of their book.

In fact, there is a clear overlap between *Action Systems* and *Jung: Revisited and Refreshed*, and each complements the other to a considerable extent. The 'action system' perceived by Donald MacKay for example is, at base, a mathematical formula which he portrays as an organism with 'mind-like processes'.

At base, however, even the concept of two simple organisms interacting with each other may be deemed 'a unit of natural action', but it is surrounded, as an 'action system'' by a most complex environment that can be described only piece-meal within a kind of 'web' or network of ideas desperately in need of organization.

Such an 'epitheoretical web' is outlined in Part Three – but only in relation to the suggested Jung-Plato paradigm. Given the resources to support its development and usage, this kind of arrangement could be very useful as a *vade mecum* or 'scratch-pad' for jotting down ephemeral ideas or trains of thought,

[In this monograph, I augment Donald MacKay's physiological aspects of mind-like processes by psychological ones in the Jungian mould, and introduce measures of subjective probability and information theory, all of which slot neatly into the exposition of Clarke with Crossland. My point is, of course, that it fits neatly with nearly everything else despite a vastly increased network of inter-relationships and their attributes and functions.

Returning to the simple relationship between two simple organisms, we find complexity relating to particle physics. For example, Roger Penrose presents a well-argued case for two *entangled* organisms (such as paramecia) to be as one via a relationship *outside space and time*.

The Axis of Scale is useful for considering this; and, if we take the material realm as the starting point (to accommodate the cilia of the paramecia), then we find that the 'oneness' of the entangled couple becomes reduced to one single relationship, i.e. one *system* in the neighbouring Realm or 'Universe' [which would be transcendental]

The implication of this is that there is a 'directness' or 'immediacy' between the material realm and the transcendental realms, and that the separate and distinct material entities are merely *'manifestations'* of one co-operative pairing of sub-principles (e.g. Yin-Yang) in *one* system at the ontological higher level (further along the axis of scale). The intermediary regions provide the mechanisms of the manifestation process.

Thus, an interface between systems appearing in one realm or level disappears at the higher level (this is one of Mattessich's metaphysical assertions or systems principles. It is not long, in such trains of thought, before the great need for an organized 'epitheoretical web' is discovered.

Neither is it long before the concept of two simple organisms in respect of living (embodied) formulae and non-living equivalents is found to be reasonable. This is soon found to be the case when we consider their taxonomic position in a table of 'Action Systems' and their parts in terms of their categorical descriptors.

To accord with MacKay's scheme of Comprehensive Reality, and for convenience, let us differentiate *Existence* into The Physical Universe and Divinity. That does not necessarily imply either the existence of Divinity or of an Environment for the physical universe, although both are likely to exist. There are more primitive dichotomies, such as the issue of why there is something rather than nothing, but that would take us into set theory.

As we take everything to be a system, then we will take the first 'categorical description' division level to be that of *Phylum*, i.e. the distinction between "Action Systems' and 'Non-Action Systems', and the following Table flows from that. The Table is loose and is for illustrative purposes only. It runs as follows:-

Level	Descriptors
Phylum	Action System = Protozoan
Class	Separate Action Information System
Order	Action *Support* Information System
Family	*Intelligent* Support Systems ('ISS's)
Genus	*Real-Time* ISS
Species	*Self-Adaptive* Real-Time ISS
Variety	*User-Analytical* R-T Self-Adaptive ISS
Strain	Living/ Non-Living/ Hybrid R-T/ S-A/ ISS

Table 1   The Increasing Complexity of Information Processing Systems

<u>Notes to Table 1</u>

1   This *seems* to imply restriction to the physical universe in some way.
2   It poses many questions as to the nature of decision-making *outside* it.
3   We are reminded that units along the Axis are powers of ten.
4   We are called upon for *Evidence* of external entities and forces.
5   These things make us focus on extra- or compacted dimensions.
6   Those lie around the Planck limits of Space and of Time (which differ).
7   This is exactly as was observed by Aristotle.

(ii) SYSTEM and USER

Table 1 illustrates the evolution of an organism's information processing capabilities – accompanying the evolution of the organism itself.   Throughout that evolution the processing of information is geared to the needs and need-satisfaction of the individual or, better, the pair of individuals in a relationship(s).

So the nature and function of the putative 'User' enter into our considerations. Jung's concept of a separate and distinct superordinate system can be ruled out from the start – especially as the 'Mind(Ego)' is now to be seen as functions of the brain. Sherrington gives us a starting point – psyche collaborates with brain, with psyche being a kind of ultimate pontifical quasi-nerve-cell.

We take the hint: the psyche is merely a pilot, determinator, or, at most, a director.   And, from our knowledge of particle physics, we can even conceive of a system of bosons piloting, determining, or directing, sets of fermions.   But, what shapes the set of bosons impressing its self upon the fermions?   We look for hidden dimensions rather than transcendence.

The organism is very likely to be in more dimensions than the four dimensions of our bodies to which we are accustomed.   Estimates of the number of additional dimensions needed range from two to infinity, but we are on happier ground in postulating that so-called 'soul-bodies' and 'spirit bodies' exist which influence our normal bodies in the Sino-Asiatic model.

Be this as it may, a search for a 'User', in hidden dimensions and fitting our description, finds a strong contender does not take us much further – He/She is just around the corne, so to speak. The notion has already been espoused by prominent Jungians of the past and the mechanics of the idea can be accepted readily, it is only the purported goal that is highly disputable. Jung claims this goal to be the Self, and nearly everyone else sees it as 'the Other'.

I refer, particularly, to the brilliant notion advanced by P.D. Ouspensky, mystic and mathematician, of Dimensional Time. This idea has been of interest to mathematicians and physicists for many decades, and it 'ticks all the boxes' in our quest for a 'User' who seems to be an amalgam of Pilot, Determinator, Director, etc., of the course to be steered along our individual life-line as we each seek to find our individual 'soul-image'.

J.B. Priestley's, *Man and Time*, is invaluable for (a) discussion of dimensional time, (b) its mathematical representation, (c) its melding with personal experience, and *above all* (d) for allowing us to perceive highly significant computer analogies.

He enable us to recognise these dimensions of Time in respect of real-time computer systems in which we have 'User time' (Simultaneity), 'Passing time', and 'Instantaneity' (wherein Potentiality is converted to Actual, thus completing Aristotle's quartet of causal forms). I will return to these aspects of dimensional time in this Part of the monograph (Part Two) and also in Part Three to show the inter-linking with other ideas.

Here, however, I bring into consideration the identities and their roles in the three dimensions of Time. So, borrowing the terminology of J.B. Priestley in relating his wartime experiences, Self 1 senses 'disturbance', Self 2 looks ahead and expects pain and, possibly, death, and Self 3 says something like the very detached 'Well, Well. Self 1 and Self 2 will soon add these things to their experience'.

The first two 'Selfs' are part of the material body but Self 3 is what might be called the psychical User – on the understanding that all three are of the physical universe. Therefore, we seek mechanisms for *interfaces* between (a) The User and the organism and (b) sets of fermions and sets of bosons, and we find what we seek.

The 'User/organism' interface is depicted by Popper and Eccles. Both in theory and in actual computer systems, within *The Self and Its Brain*. The interface between fermions and bosons is the one discussed by Danah Zohar (and David Hodgson) which actually exists in living tissue (under certain conditions) The match is very close in real-time computer systems and in the extra dimensions introduced by the Hind yogic tradition.

More details can be found either in the books cited or in Part Three (e.g. under 'Models'), but it may be that models of all interfaces – inside or outside the physical universe – can be modelled by material constructs. This rather supports Polkinghorne's assertion that if any 'outside' entities influence and affect us in the material world, then we should be able to detect it scientifically.

The axis of scale, with its 'units' of orders of magnitude suggests otherwise – especially to particle physicists with their predeliction for atom-smashing. In regard of the Sino-Asiatic model, cogent models can be provided in terms of electromagnetic 'coils', piano keyboards, beads in an abacus, and even clothes on a clothes-line. (see Part Three)

(iii) THE IMPOSITION OF CONSTRAINTS

Still within the physical universe and 'normal' four-dimensional space-time, we can conceive of two sets of constraints. The first set is within the biological stream (Jung called it turmoil) and the second is that imposed upon the organism, as a whole, as a mixed aggregate of specifications of performance, resources, priorities, weaponry, size, shape, and so on.

In the conjectured extra dimensions afforded by the Hindu yogic tradition or, more widely, the 'Sino-Asiatic model, the parameters of a 'soul-body' and a 'spirit body' are given specifically. The former is supposed to follow the organismal material body, and the latter is ovoid in shape. This is described well by Hiroshi Motoyama.

More detailed and technical limited constraints are imposed by the operating system and its two primary suites of software at the deeper evolutionary levels indicated by Table 1. The 'operating system', for example, is that provided by the basic levels of the 'Triune brain' (see Livesey; and Part Three) and all is analogous to the real-time computer systems about which Donald MacKay and I write (separately and independently).

The operating system of an operational organism of this kind is centred upon the two main tasks of (a) maintaining the smooth and efficient running of the mechanistic organism and (b) to provide helpful, processed information for its User. To do this in a real-time situation the key function is probably the operation of a cyclic scanning of a rota of program suites, i.e. Processes. Two essential features are an *interrupt system* (which can interrupt the cyclic scan) and a *vectored priority ordering system*.

Of the program suites and processes within the rota being scanned, two essential and major *areas* of software are the so-called 'System' software and the 'Application' software. This division of labour corresponds loosely to the mechanistic and smooth running of the organism and to the dealing with contingencies arising in the outside world, i.e. the environment.

Among the *program suites* being scanned, there is one that is both extremely important and extremely powerful – it is called the *Supervisor* and it is also extremely large. It has been mistaken for the Command element, but it is only a huge program suite. [If Ernest Kent's assertion is correct, then all kinds of monistic consequences ensue; but mathematical Platonism, coupled with Comprehenive Reality, can accommodate such an eventuality.]

One most important constraint imposed by the operating system, therefore, is that of keeping a balance between the two processes within acceptable limits within its powers, e.g. allocation of resources, priorities, etc., and it has the power to suspend processes if necessary. In humans, the conditions of Extraversion and Introversion will obtain should the *balance* be broken.   I repeat that this is a loose description because computer systems vary according to any number of requirements.

There is even more complexity in these region, however, because deep in the heart of the operating system there lies a piece of mechanism that has only a dual function and is called a 'central processing unit'.   Its dual function is that of Machine Logic and Control.

We cannot go beyond the machine logic – this is the level at which individual program 'orders' (i.e. instructions and addresses) are broken down into pieces and each piece is translated into a hardware operation *at the same time*.   In other words (those of Aristotle) *potential* is concerted into *actual*.

Three levels can be recognized in a hierarchy or 'triage' – each operates under constraints.   There is the Supervisor program suite (tens of thousands of subroutines) which is pure software.   The operating system is a mixture of hardware and software; and the central processing unit (as it is called) is pure hardware.   All obtains within one organism which is built from the most elementary building blocks, such as clocks, timers, 'flag', markers, etc.

Without attributing any significance to it, it is noteworthy that triages obtain in the physical universe, some of which are shown in Table Two:-

Leptons and Quarks	Causal Plane	CPU	time Three
Bosons and Fermions	Astral Plane	OS	time Two
Atoms	Material Plane	Program	time One

Table 2   Triages in the Physical Universe

This set excludes Christianity but includes levels identified within the Sino-Asiatic model.   Levels from Christianity can be associated with those portrayed - as is shown by Hiroshi Motoyama.   A striking feature of the set is that it does not reflect any 'great chain of being' (Lovejoy) or 'chain of Command', but it *does* reflect 'a great hierarchy of being'.

It seems, indeed, that the extra dimensions posited by the Hindu yogic tradition enable us – as we investigate further along the axis of scale – to visualize 'bodies' that may lack Command power but have much *Situational* power.

This kind of power obtains in the triage of 'Spirit Body', 'Soul Body', and 'Manifested (Material) Body'.   In other words, the 'Spirit Body' gives a specification for the 'Soul Body', and the 'Soul Body' gives the specification for the material 'Woman' or 'Man' (following Yin and Yan).   It is not too difficult to perceive these in terms 'Ideal Forms' as 'specifications'.

The cross-correlation in Table 2 would not have been possible under Jung's concept of Personality, Mind, and Ego, being features of a non-material system.   The encephalization of these features, therefore, has a very significant effect (for the better) on Jungian theory.

(iv)) CONSEQUENCES OF ENCEPHALIZATION

The re-locating of Jungian Personality, Mind and Ego from a postulated non-material system to a purely material computer system, and thence, to a naturally evolved brain has consequences far beyond the superficial. They are, almost literally, *seismic* - almost the whole system of thought, one might say, comes crashing to the ground. But, this is exactly what was needed. The Jungian system is elevated to a prestigious significance.

The triages mentioned in the last few paragraphs are almost as nothing in comparison with the 'hardening up' of numerous vague concepts and the provision of supporting computer models. The additional 'weight of evidence' secured is massive (discussed in Part One). And, Part Three contains entries which give exact and very plausible (and much needed) meanings and roles to the Animus/Anima as navigator/ pilot/ leader/ steersman/ director matching precisely with Timothy O'Neill's interpretation of the Animus/ Anima.

Another vague bundle of concepts produced by Jung has to do with the 'carrying over' of knowledge upon dying – in a military computer system this procedure is almost word-for-word as it is described by Jung – and more. I have already referred to Ideal Forms as 'specifications', and these pertain very much to an amalgam of 'Operating Characteristics', 'Design Requirements', etc., etc., set by and for future Users.

(v) NEW APPROACHES TO MODELLING

The name, 'Ouspensky', crops up continually, and in the most respectable and learned circles. His 'intuitional' logic joins with deductive logic and inductive logic to provide yet another Triage. And, in Part Three I have assembled – for example and for use with Jungian theory – a 'Notional Epitheoretical Web' – which gives us insight not only into thought processes but also to their particular potential for analysis and synthesis.

I refer to the intuitional logic that could lie within the bounds of evolutionary psychology but outside the limits of the other two forms of logic. These, of course, depend upon knowledge, and 'Primum Organum', 'Organum Secundus', and 'Tertium Organum' form a triage of means of acquiring knowledge.

For example, had Plato and Aristotle possessed our present-day knowledge of Computer Systems, Set Theory, the Transfinite, etc., they might well have arrived at the same conclusions regarding Causality, Metempsychosis and Ideal Forms, but Tertium Organum, i.e. Intuitional Logic, enables us to surmise their trains of thought in retrospect and to make preditions that can be tested.

In such respects, I can give an example from my own experience of the latter, which is pertinent and cogent in regard of prediction. During discussion with a friend, I had communicated the notion of Platonic 'elective' or 'eclectic' affinities having identical neural structures powered and shaped respectively by Yin and by Yang. This would reflect that they were 'contained' within the "Spirit Body" outside the physical universe.

To exemplify this, I used the simile of a clothes line bearing light garments typical of ladies and heavy duty garments, such as heavy dungaries, for reprenting the male. The former would flutter in light breezes and both sets would flutter in heavy winds, thus providing different patterns. But, we soon realized that this was unsatisfactory.

So, after a period of reflection, the thought came to me that the bi-polarity of magnetism might provide a better model, and I provided an 'improved model' in which the same neural circuits would give different patterns if they acted as solenoids distributed within the brains.

Purely out of curiosity, and not expecting to find an entry, I looked up 'solenoid' in a scientific dictionary – and there it was! The entry read: 'The organization of nucleosomes and space regions into a solenoid coil, containing 6-7 nucleosomes per turn, with a diameter of 30mm.' The heading was 'Solenoid Model', and it was on page 1112 of *'Chambers Dictionary of Science and Technology' 2007*.

This mechanization of the Association of Ideas makes Freud's 'Free Association' not merely more soundly based but also more *plausible*. *It* does the same for Jung's notion of a 'complex' of ideas. In fact, it makes the concept 'only to be expected' within 'mechanistic embodiment'.

This notion of 'prediction' can be extended back to the ideologies of Plato and Aristotle. For example, the rhetorical question can be posed, 'Would not Plato have used the simile of *the Cave* had he had today's knowledge (conception) of a '*Life Force beamed (projected) through mathematical Platonism to produce manifestations of Men and Women?*' Or, the computer equivalent; or Jung's 'diving suit'?

It is but a short step from these issue to the similar matters of Mysticism and Clairvoyance (not to mention Extra-Sensory Perception). The coverage given by William Johnston, J.B. Priestley, and even John Polkinghorne suffices – amid a great many of equal status.

Figure 2 gives a loose outline of the putative Jung-Plato paradigm. Its simplicity and aptness is in striking contrast to the 'baroque grandeurs' pictured by Jung of the vistas imagined by his 'psychic eye'. But, then, Jung conceived of Personality pertaining to a psychic body, and not to any material 'body' – be it brain or computer.

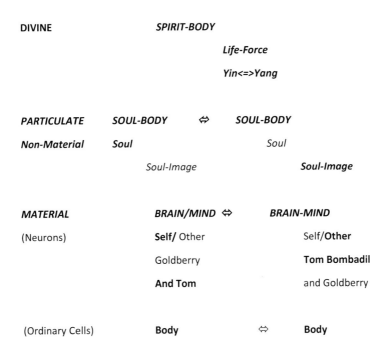

DIVINE		SPIRIT-BODY		
		Life-Force		
		Yin<=>Yang		
PARTICULATE	*SOUL-BODY*	⇔	*SOUL-BODY*	
Non-Material	*Soul*		*Soul*	
	Soul-Image		*Soul-Image*	
MATERIAL	*BRAIN/MIND* ⇔		*BRAIN-MIND*	
(Neurons)	**Self/** Other		Self/**Other**	
	Goldberry		**Tom Bombadil**	
	And Tom		and Goldberry	
(Ordinary Cells)	**Body**	⇔	**Body**	

Figure 2   Sino-Asiatic Affinitive Relationship along the Axis of Scale

Notes.

1. Jung believed that 'the Other' was entirely fictive and stochastic.
2. This conflicts with his concept of soul-image (Munroe, p. 560-2).
3. He believed that the goal of psychic development is the Self.
4. He saw the Animus/ Anima as an accumulation of features of real women casually acquired over aeons of time and building up a real image of a fictive woman that could be disposed of after use.
5. This process culminated in the fictive 'Anticipated Whole Other' which was ued and then discarded.
6. In the J-P paradigm, the A/A is a _real_ Psychagogue/ Guide.
7. Figure 2 reflects the possibility of modelling in the Complex Plane.

(vi) EXTRAVERSION and INTROVERSION

I have shown how the processes of a real-time military computer system serve to explain and illustrate our own everyday experience.   Lying behind (or below) the dichotomy between Extraversion and Introversion, however, there is a singular feature that goes far deeper and wider, and which ramifies out into every aspect of our being – bringing everyday experience into the realm of mathematics.

I refer again to the notion of 'dimensional time' advanced by P.D Ouspensky, championed by J.B. Priestley, converted into mathematical form by P.G. Bennett, and enthusiastically espoused by leaders in the Jungian fraternity of the time. As I have explained, Introversion tends to emphasize *system* processes and extraversion focusses upon environmental events and entities – and this involves the time-dependencies of these sets of processes.

Broadly speaking, system processes operate at *speeds* different from those of application processes. The former may be 'on-line', but the latter are 'real-time'. Being irritated by Jung's use of the blanket term, 'Unconscious', I choose often to use the hierarchy of mental levels, i.e. subconscious, *'periconscious'*, conscious, and superconscious.

In this area, the computer analogies prove to be extremely useful in the wider field of experience. And this is because they show how different processes operate at different speeds and are called into service by the efforts of the operating system and the Supervisor suite of programs working together.

A newcomer to the deepest levels of machine code programming often finds this quite perplexing. The crux of the matter lies in the fact that while the operating systems scans and executes its rota of programs in *machine* or *computer time*, the application programs operate at a very much faster rate.

The difference in speeds is really mind-boggling; and if one imagines the 'computer time' in terms of the hour intervals marked on a clock-face, then (even in the 1950s) the time intervals for application programs could not be marked because they would be so small.

This is not all, however, because it is now possible to delineate three 'dimensions of Time *at right angles to each other* as was conjectured by Ouspensky, Priestley, and Bennett. At the User level there is *simultaneity*. Computer time runs linearly as '*passing time*'. At the basic level whereat the program code is converted to hardware operations, there is *Immediacy* or *Instantaneity*.

It is noteworthy that this phenomenon of *Instantaneity* shown in computers (and conjectured in humans) may well apply to protozoa. Roger Penrose makes a not inconsiderable case, re the lower animals with no neurons, for the operation of cytoskeletal quantum effects giving non-locality.

(vii) JUDGEMENT and PERCEPTION

With the Jungian modes of Judgement and Perception, i.e. the 'four functions', I can illustrate a specific and precise match of the warship's functions with those identified as human mental functions. Their descriptions are variously from Ruth Munroe, David Cox, and Anthony Storr.

(a) <u>Sensation</u>

concerns the present, the *NOW*.   It tells us that a thing *IS*.   A thing is either *PRESENT* or *ABSENT*.

(b) <u>Intuition</u>

Is concerned with the *POTENTIAL* of the thing and its possibilities in the *FUTURE,* judged from its past.   It seeks to establish the thing's *SIGNIFICANCE.*

(c) <u>Feeling</u>

addresses *VALUES* with regard to *POSSIBLE ACTION.*   Is it to be *ACCEPTED* or *REJECTED?*   Is it *AGREEABLE* or *DISAGREEABLE?*   Is it *GOOD* or is it *BAD?*

(d) <u>Thinking</u>

conducts a rational analysis of WHAT the thing *IS*.   It IDENTIFIES the thing.   It *CATEGORIZES* the thing.

<u>NOTES</u>

(1) Exact parallels with these processes relate to a warship's radar processing and, usually, to a 'screen'.   In sequence, loosely, the radar *Detects* that a target is present.   It then A*ssesses* (e.g. Safety/ Danger) from the target's attitude, course, speed, size, height, etc., whether further investigation is necessary.   Having *evaluated (e.e. Friend/ Foe)* the target's *significance* the 'thing' can be left alone, investigated more fully, or shot down.

(2) It is noteworthy that such almost impeccable analogies go very much against the grain of Anthony Storr's comment that their identification by Jung is his 'least valuable contribution' (pp. 77-9).   Dr. Storr (one of my 'source authors) remarked, further, that the 'quaternity of the four functions has been discarded by all exept the most dedicated Jungians, and is...little used by them' (!).

(3) Jung deserves praise for his perception.   He discerned the four *natural* functions, but allocated them wrongly to the non-material psyche when, in fact, they are part of the biological turmoil that he so despised.   This, together with the 'natural quaternion', is part and parcel of the Mind(Ego) encephalization.   In short, the process endorses Ruth Munroe's remark that Jung becomes more acceptable when he returns closer to Freud.

(viii) The Collective Unconscious, Archetypes, Relational Discernment

(a) *Relationships*

Ruth Munroe's comment about the drawing together of Freudian and Jungian ideas carries over into the notion of collective unconsciousness and standard, immediately recognizable and enforceable, protocols, formats, channels for information transfer, and so on.

I will refrain from quoting her, but I will condense her opinions and correlate them with my own wherever and whenever possible in this section. Let me say from the start that my analogies between Jungian theory and a warship in these matters find favour with an unknown number of Jungians. [I know this because my Establishment (ASWE), wishing to safeguard Security, took the precaution of check out my thesis with Jungian authorities.]

Be this at it may, Dr. Munroe and I share a distaste for Jung's excessive fondness for the Mandala symbol. In essence, she drains this symbol and archetype of all the significance awarded it by Jung, and places *archetypes,* as a whole, at a 'bio-social' level.

Although I agree largely with this, I pay heed to the thoughts of William James, Walter Mons, Teilhard de Chardin, and countless others, and give credence to the possibility of a higher level which is either 'psycho-social' or 'super-social' and touches upon normative and/or deontic levels. We need possible recourse to these levels in order to deal successfully with 'the social Leviathan'.

I concur, also, with Ruth Munroe's interpretation of the Mandala as a variable form of 'body-image' representation. Likewise, we seem to think alike about the four functions being down at the 'biological' level. The four functions may be pretty basic – as I have shown – but they are operating at social levels fashioned by the brain/mind.

Lower than the human brain in evolution, we can think more in terms of the kind of mechanism suggested by Roger Penrose, and, with the human brain at its best, we are up into the 'superconscious' pictured by William James, and others.

The concept of a non-material 'collective unconscious' is a difficult one in its own right – because it is, very largely, conjectural and fragmented, and very difficult to examine by experimental methods. The warship analogy offers a considerable number of convincing and cogent models.

Understanding of the concept really needs specialist input from somewhere. Ruth Munroe was a psychologist (of Freudian inclinations) especially requested to make a survey of the majors schools of psychoanalytic thought (from that level). I labour the point, because it is very clear that an epitheoretic approach was needed.

In my opinion, Dr. Munroe did a pretty good job – within those limitations. She set out her terms of reference and gave definitions of her meaning – when she could. However, with the *collective unconscious*, she was forced to fall back upon an unusually large number of quotations (for which she apologised) and a few personal and hesitant conjectures about Jung's meaning.

She was, however, neither a psychiatrist nor a therapist. David Stafford-Clark <u>was</u> a psychiatrist, and a Freudian, to boot. In *Psychiatry Today* (pp. 154-5) he describes Jung's 'remarkable conception' and comments that for a student of psychopathology and psychodynamics it is an 'indispensable field for exploration'.

As the merest outline of what Jung had in mind, David Stafford-Clark makes an illuminating stab at outlining Jung's construct. He portrays mountain ranges rising up from a plateau, with individual mountains rising up from them – each with its 'peak' of consciousness.   This is graphic only up to a point – beyond that it is static, solid, and infertile.

There is no need to quote Ruth Munroe on this because Stafford-Clark's 'mountain range' analogy and the ISS's 'warship' analogy are both illustrative of the fact that the 'world' is nothing but an ordered bundle of relationships – of varying orders and degrees (i.e. categories) manifested in the material realm.

The 'poles' of each relationship have counterbalancing effects upon each other, with the joint subjective aim of enhancing the relationship and the entity within which it is mechanistically embedded.   The Sino-Asiatic Model provides 'bodies' by which this can take place, i.e. the equivalents of the Christian 'Soul-Body' and 'Spirit-Body'.

(b) Archetypes, Ideal Forms, and Discernment

Several things follow from this, but the most obvious is, perhaps, that *Archetypes* and *Ideal Forms* are radically different from each other although both feature in noesis. Archetypes are very much the product of the human mind and they serve either offensive or defensive purposes in a war against the hordes of foes within the social Leviathan.

Ideal Forms, on the other hand, although stemming from the Brain/ Mind, are concepts serving the pursuit of *Perfection*.   Whereas archetypes may be conjured up from the various generators in the brain, ideal forms are things that have to be reached out for in constructs of the Brain/ Mind.

The 'generators' to which I referred are those physiological systems depicted by Donald MacKay, but the 'searching out' processes seems to come from a higher functional system.   I have in mind (i) the difference between Jung's concepts of Intuition and Feeling, and (ii) my own experience.

Although this seems to be to Jung's credit (apart from the displacement), it does not obviate the gross error made by the early Jungians who carried Jung's fanatical Individualism into Ouspenskian fields, so to speak (see Priestley; Rucker).

P.D. Ouspensky was an out-and-out Relationist.   He was, also, one the greatest philosophers of the 20th century.   In *Tertium Organum* mathematics enters and pervades the field of philosophy – so writes, in 1922, the author of the Introduction to the book, Claude Bragdon (pp. 1-6).   For our purposes, however, there are two very special features about Ouspensky.

The first feature is that specifies the third element in a relationship, namely the relationship itself (pp. 236).   And, he does so in a special way that is completely within the Sino-Asiatic model and the Jung-Plato paradigm.   Regretting that the axioms of *Tertium Organum* cannot be formulated in human language, Ouspensky does his best by taking the axioms of Aristotle as a model.

He expresses the principal axiom of intuitive logic in three alternative ways wherein exactly the same meaning prevails.   They are:-

A is both A and Not-A.

or

Everything is both A and Not-A.

or

Everything is All.

He then, immediately, points out the absurdity of this triage in the logic of Aristotle and of Bacon

However, the importance and the pertinence of Ouspensky's point appears if we make the substitution of 'Self' for 'A', whereupon 'B' becomes 'Not-Self' (or 'Other'). We recognise that this is the dichotomy cited as the basis of the Jungian 'problematic'; and, equally quickly, we perceive what is missing. The third element, i.e. the 'relationship', per se, is missing and belongs to other dimensions.

The ideas of higher logic are *inexpressible in concepts*, says Peter Ouspensky. To master the fundamental principles of higher *logic* we have to master the fundamentals of the understanding of a *space of higher dimensions* (p. 237). Then, he explains and expands upon this.

To follow this, I refer to Rudy Rucker's book, *The fourth Dimension and how to get there*, wherein Rucker cites and quotes from Peter Ouspensky's works. On pages 58-9, Rucker explains that Ouspensky saw the 'fourth dimension' not only as a spatial concept but also as a type of consciousness, and awareness of greater complexities and higher unities.

For him, says Rucker, the mathematical study of the fourth dimension led quite naturally to a belief in the teachings of Mysticism [as we have just seen]. Rucker is suggesting that perhaps we ourselves are, in some very real sense, beings of *more than three dimensions*.

Rucker then explicates of this by suggesting that higher space can be viewed as a 'background of connective tissue tying together the world's most diverse phenomena'. Also, that 'if one moves toward higher and higher conceptions, one is tending toward some ideal "Superspace" in which everything - near and far, past and future, big and small, real and imagined – is together in some great unity'.

Today, more than a century later, we can understand fully his point; and, moreover, we have a number of 'triages' to which his principal axiom can be applied. But, again, for our purposes there is an equally important precept in *Tertium Organum* which (on its own account) places Ouspensky with modern masters of psychodynamics, such as Ethel Spector Person and Rollo May.

(c) *The Agent of Change*

I refer to Ouspensky on *Love*. Because his words are relevant to my comments on Jungian functions of *intuiting* and *Feeling*, I quote Ouspensky's paragraph (p. 153) in full:

Love unfolds in a human being trai traits of his which he never new in himself. In love there is much both of the Stone Age and of the Witches' Sabbath. By anything less than love many men cannot be induced to commit a crime, to be guilty of a treason, to reanimate in themselves such feelings as they thought to have killed out long ago. In love is hidden an infinity of egoism, vanity and selfishness. Love is the potent force that tears off all masks, and men who run away from love do so in order that they may preserve their masks.

It is the final sentence that interests me. It does so because for Ouspensky – through personal love, which Jung eschews – one achieves exactly the 'unmasking' which Jung (and others) says is essential in facing up to the endless run of ethical decisions which one has to make in ordinary daily life.

In ten pages (149-157) P.D. Ouspensky writes baldly and knowingly about men's attitude to Love. He echoes the thoughts of Plato in saying that

Only he who can see considerably beyond *the facts* discerns love's real meaning; and it is possible to illumine these very facts by the light of that which lies behind them.

His continuance of that theme echoes William Johnston, Ethel Person and Rollo May. Ouspensky points out that he who *is* able to see beyond the 'facts' begins to discern much of 'newness' *in love and through love*. And, here we begin to appreciate mystical union, mystical merger, indwelling, and the *mystical knowledge (clairvoyance)* that comes with them.

(d) Relational Discernment

We can contain all the features mentioned in this section (viii) within the Jung-Plato paradigm. Donald MacKay's Comprehensive Reality, Mathematical Platonism, the Hindu yogic tradition, and particle physics, all combine to provide for a relationship between two variables (manifested in the material level) to be represented as a bivariate mathematical function capable of discerning the Good and working towards freedom from karma at that level.

We may surmise that the function intuits, and has a feeling for, the Good through the smooth continuity of its progression as a 'world line'. Any flaw in its performance produces a change in the smooth continuity, which ultimately leads to chaos and confusion. The Good is therefore as Plato saw it – an ideal form – which has to be discerned, but the 'action' takes place in the material level against the long 'limbs' of the social Leviathan.

It is worthy of note that Ludwig von Bertalanffy sees the human organism in much the same light. He reduces it to a set of differential equations - see pages 53-94 of *General System Theory*, wherein he addresses System Concepts in Elementary Mathematical Consideration. Speaking *very* loosely, perhaps we could consider 'relational discernment' as some form of mathematical integration or, even, differentiation.

To formulate the model we just need to transform Ouspensky's 'A' into 'Self' whereupon 'NOT- A' becomes the 'Other and a relationship between two entangled entities leaps into being in a different dimension – as in Figure 2. This is not possible in the worlds of Aristotle and of Bacon, but I have constructed the Figure to illustrate how a simple folding of the page along a vertical axis could introduce, for example, an orthogonal complex plane.

In relation to Jungian theory, two features are very puzzling. First, how on earth did Jung not see this, in view of his two functions of *Intuition* and *Feeling*? Second, why could not Danah Zohar, with her scheme of 'Relational Holism', see that all the wave-functions producing her pantheistic 'I' must (surely?) be ordered and arranged according to some deontic and normative scheme.

(e) Communications (or, Personal Love *is* Cosmogonic)

I feel a need to add to the thoughts of Ouspensky, and of Freud, and of Jung, over this matter. Each , of them (in my opinion, wrongly) associates Love, personified as Eros, with all kinds of vicissitudes which are nothing to do with Love. Even the early and classical Greeks identified an 'uneasy' relationship between Ares and Aphrodite.

The relationship is 'uneasy' because it can be so easily misconceived and misrepresented – perhaps never so much as it is today. Still talking in terms of demi-gods, it can be posited that Mammon was introduced and made grandiose over the last hundred years or so, wherein 'economies with the truth' and the wider dissemination of falsehoods became almost 'standard practice' by the social Leviathan.

During this time, profit became explicable in terms of ' justifiable gratification of desire' for Self regardless of Other. We have it in Jung's own words: The goal of psychic development is the Self. And, the 'Jungian problematic' has remained so ever since – until the interpretation of the Anima/ Animus was corrected by Timothy O'Neill.

However, there *do* remain certain areas of Mysticism to be tied into the picture, and Jung was perfectly correct in relating such things as psychagogues, visions, personifications to personal experience – it was his *interpretation* of his personal experiences that erred. And so, in the Appendix, I include my own personal experiences of that ilk, of which my attempts at analysis result in nothing that cannot be accounted for by the Jung-Plato paradigm.

By this I mean that Mystical Love, Union, Merger, and Indwelling - as presented by William Johnston and by Rollo May – are all part of Donald MacKay's Comprehensive Reality in accordance with Evolutionary Psychology in a physical universe containing a half-a-dozen or so 'extra' dimensions (as in the Sino-Asiatic model.

Many factors contribute to this. Heuristic learning is tied to emotion (Livesey). Jung's hierarchy of Eve, Helen, Mary, and Sapientia, obtains. The Animus/ Anima is real and not fictive.   Many forms of Information exist.   Lay mysticism is part of the physical universe.   Spiritual beings exist in the physical universe and the triune brain is part of this. Mechanistic embodiment prevails, and so on.

(ix) Encephalization of Command

MacKay's mechanization of 'mind-like processes', in effect, includes the mechanistic embodiment of the Command function.   He includes two functionaries, the '*Agent*' and the '*Determinator*', within his embodied formula; and this, in the context of mathematical Platonism allied with the Sino-Asiatic idiom, is sufficient to provide Comprehensive Reality.

In addition to following Ruth Munroe's desideratum of 'returning' towards Freud, this is consistent and coherent with Artificial Intelligence and with ever-advancing military operational software – and with an ever-increasing sensitivity to the needs of Security!

This movement has great profundity and great depth; and, in a nutshell, it leads us to basic considerations of noesis and praxeology, i.e. cognition and decision-making.   In other words, through heuristic learning and relational memory, etc., it gives considerable support to the notion of Evolutionary Psychology.

We can even surmise that it affords anawers to the fundamental philosophical question, 'Why is there something rather than nothing?'.   A putative answer is manifest: it is ' To allow Choice and to enable Free-Will'.   This is not facile.   For example, Donald MacKay posited, in *Freedom in a Mechanistic Universe*, that this gives an individual the freedom to change – to become different from what he is.

It may not be possible to discuss military matters very deeply, but we can exemplify the movement in other areas, such as chess.   The fact that chess-playing programs can beat human world champions with ease cannot be swept aside with platitudes or canards about size and capacity.   When concepts of heuristic learning etc., are included it becomes clear that size, heuristic learning, and *pattern matching*, will one day make the computer (software) unbeatable.

To this notion, we can also add the capability of 'weighing' the evidential value (per context and theme) of propositions.   This, too, is based upon the most fundamental concept of choice and free-will.   For example, we cannot conceive of 'nothing' without introducing 'something', e.g. the 'empty set' in set theory.   Or, the principle (in process philosophy) that an 'occasion of experience' cannot exist on its own

Thus, from such ideas, we intuit that the functions of Agency and of Command are drawing ever closer, but never identical – otherwise thay would represent an automaton. It *does* seem possible that one fundamental piece of rationality may be a universal, namely a need to distinguish between 'Self' and 'Other'.

At this point, it seems advisable to offer definitions or, at least, examples.   Failing this, then a statement of the situation seems called for.   Therefore, I start with Christian allegory as it is advanced by C.S. Lewis.   Adding to my earlier references to *That Hideous*

Strength, which seems so well to illustrate our position today, I refer to a discussion being held between Christian apologists, Dr. Dimble and his wife.

The former remarks that, at any time in history, one can perceive a distinction between past, when there was more 'elbow-room' and contrasts weren't so sharp, and future, where there is even less room for indecision and choices are more momentous (pp. 173-4). Mrs. Dimble might have been reading Jung on ethical decisions, because she refers to Browning's line: 'Life's business being just the terrible choice'.

Agreeing with his wife, Dimble makes a further point, to the effect that: 'Minds get more spiritual, matter more material. Poetry and prose draw farther apart'. In the sense that the qualities assigned by Jung to the 'spiritual' are proving to belong to material entities, and matter has an underlayer of particles, this holds good today. As does the distinction between poetry and prose, which is partly because language is being obliterated.

But I cite this because it begs the bringing-in of other knowledge, such as the subject-matter of this monograph. And, over this, I return to Ruth Munroe. A dictionary of philosophy (edited by Blackburn) gives on (page 357) the definition of 'soul' as: 'The immaterial "I" that possesses conscious experience, controls passion, desire and action, and maintains a perfect identity from birth (or before) to death (or after)'.

This definition serves (as well as any other *existing* definition) to illustrate my point. My point being that Ruth Munroe was not able to form a reliable opinion on the collective unconscious without using many quotations, but she <u>did </u>furnish the seeds of its understanding – some seventy years in advance.

She did this in a very simple way by repeating a number of times, in close juxtaposition – the *'I' of common parlance* and the *'soul-image'*. The former term she equates with *'ego-consciousness'*, and the second term with the *'Animus/ Anima'*. The distinction is central to the Sino-Asiatic model and to the Jung-Plato paradigm which embraces it.

In this area Jung seems to have become somewhat confused. In Part Three, it can be seen that Jung, and some of his followers, misunderstood, or misrepresented, the Sino-Asiatic model of Yin and Yang. Ruth Munroe takes Jung at his words in her representation of the soul-image, which I try to show in Figure 2.

In short, the *Anima* works upon and with the feminine part of a Man's psyche. The *Animus* operates on and through the masculine part of a woman's psyche. A Man-Woman relationship is therefore a joint effort towards re-union – as is shown in many mythical or legendary relationships.

The Odysseus –Penelope myth is an archetypal example of this. Odysseus, although enslaved by a sorceress, wept on the shore because he was prevented from pursuing re-union with his Beloved. He <u>knew</u> that she would be keeping her end up. Penelope strove mightily to stave off her suitors, <u>*knowing*</u> that Odysseus would get back to her if he possibly could.

In a taxonomy of Relationships, this would, perhaps, be classified as 'affinitive search and re-union'. Others, say Lancelot and Guinevere, might be labelled 'affinitive love botched by lacked of restraint' (Orpheus and Euridice might be a variation upon the same theme). And so on.

All of this squares with assertions by top-flight scientists that the only existents in the physical universe are relations and fields, and there is a mathematically beautiful simplicity and symmetry about it. It makes sense out of nonsense.

The 'Anticipated Whole Other', for example, becomes a concept completely related to Reality, rather than fictive, meaningless, and disposable. The notion of individuation then becomes keyed into the logical progression already nominated by Jung as 'Eve, Helen, Mary, and Sapientia, which is in accord with mystical experience and communication.

It can be seen, therefore, that Dr.Ruth Munroe merits full recognition for her contribution to MacKay's Comprehensive Realism. Through her analysis we recognise that powers, commonly attributed to a 'soul' are being found in the material world, while other powers are whittled down to issues of pilotage and leadership attributable to 'extra dimensions' in the physical universe – all within one 'n-dimensional' organism that is the mechanistic embodiment of a mathematical formula.

(x) Normative and Deontic Factors

Following from this, questions of Free Will and Qualities of Command arise. In Comprehensive Realism, Donald MacKay allows an individual to have only the freedom to be 'different from what he is', and MacKay presents a context for this quite similar to that drawn by the poet, Omar Khayyam. In other words, he allows a 'character in a story' to depart from 'the script' – see his *Freedom of Action in a Mechanistic Universe*.

It is noteworthy that C.S. Lewis adopted a similar approach by conceiving of individuals judging whether or not somebody is 'in their story'. [This proves to be a helpful decision-making concept in real, everyday life] A moment's thought about this results in the opinion that this is culture dependent, and I return to the Ancient Greeks who were pagan and polytheistic.

I first encountered Odysseus almost exactly eighty years ago, in the story of his escaping from Polyphemus. I was only seven years old, but it made me feel vaguely uneasy, and today I can fully accept that deceit and guile lie at the heart of warfare, but I have quite strong doubts as to their employment in everyday life. Although it was employed in warfare, I still have reservations about the Trojan Horse.

The social Leviathan employs such devices in its attack upon us, and I believe that complete and utter honesty – within the bounds of current attitudes to decency and legality – should be our best ambition. As both Ouspensky and Jung aver, we should strip ourselves bare in our understandings of ourselves. Ouspensky, of course, saw clearly that personal Love achieves this, Jung had no such weapon to make use of.

And so, I come to Plato and 'the Good'. The early Greeks of the time of Odysseus and Penelope had codes of honour – according to their own lights. They separated Sex from Love – quite reasonably - but they had little time for ethical decisions. If they wanted something that could be taken honourably), then they took it. For them, fortune favoured the strong or the wily.

Should they fail in achieving what they wanted, they metaphorically shrugged their shoulders or made a sacrifice to the appropriate divinity. For example, the ten years that Odysseus spent in trying to get back to Penelope was largely his own fault – he should not have offended Poseidon, the father of Polythemus.

Odysseus had no choice in being a 'sex-slave' to Calypso – she was an enchantress [imagination boggles at the notion] – but a 'sub-committee' of lesser Gods caused pressure to borne upon Poseidon, and Calypso had little choice but to free him.

The early Greeks, however, were no fools. They differentiated between body and Psyche ('soul'), and they were beginning to associate thought with the material body by believing that thought and information-processing were associated with the function of breathing. The triage of Classical Greek philosophers - Socrates, Plato, and Aristotle – changed all the atmosphere of polytheism.

Aristotle and Bacon, respectively, introduced Deductive and Inductive logi, and recently Peter Ouspensky tidied things up by introducing Tertium Oranum, i.e. Intuitive logic. Through Ouspensky, we can today conceive more easily what Plato, all that time ago, meant by 'the Good'. It is an ideal form that hs to be 'intuited' and 'felt'.

The Good incorporates therefore perfect forms which can only be approximated in the physical universe. This hardly matters, because there is no uncertainty in mathematical Platonism – only imprecision. The amount of Truth, therefore, in a situation is a matter of degree, and of context and theme.

Thus, we find along the axis of scale various bounds and limits to measurement and perception. And, also, at base under Whitehead's process philosophy, various 'principles of limitation'. All of which pertain to the 'subjective aim' of an organism that is, essentially, a wave-form, sweeping through the mathematical framework or 'screen', that produces 'manifestations' of men and women as in shadows on a cave wall.

(xi) The Warship Analogy

In this section – despite the heading – I treat both human being and warship as 'Action Systems' possessing 'Intelligent Support Systems'. The examples I give are in terms of the warship analogy because they are, so to speak, *factual*, whereas their corresponding human attributes and functions are not *so* clearly factual.

Sometimes the symptoms are the same, but is it is conjecture that the underlying mechanisms are the same. Ludwig von Bertalanffy and Richard Mattessich might well say directly that they are isomorphs, but I aim to be more cautious.   Especially so, because we are dealing with varying *levels* within the physical universe.

A further feature is that the discussion relates to my personal systems experience which knits so well with Donald MacKay's Comprehensive Realism.   That *experience* enables me to view, and to comment upon, certain aspects of Jungian theory – psychagogues, psychic input, psychic imperatives and 'hints' from the unconscious and so on.

Such experiences are described in the Appendix, but they are not only apposite at this point in my thesis, but also explanatory and, in my opinion, *significant*.   So, in the following few paragraphs I beg leave to set out the way I became able to make a dedication to my psychagogue and Anima, Rosamunda, with whom I have conversed.

I became aware of intuitions and feelings, seemingly 'external' to my ego-awareness, and apparently 'superior' to my rational mental equipment, in 'middle age'. That is to say, when my children had left home, when I had ben given recognition for a number of papers, and when I had reached the highest level open to anyone whose work was (almost) pure science, in the sense that it was not contaminated with administration and, hence, politics.

In short, as did Jung, I came to realize the accuracy of 'sudden decisive impulses' and 'hints from the unconscious'.   As did Jung, also, I became willing to trust the intuitions and feelings without recourse to their origins.   *Unlike* Jung, however, I did not ascribe them to any psychagogue.   If I thought about such input at all, I thought it was perhaps some *superconscious* part of *me*.

Then, well into retirement, I learned about the Hindu yogic tradition and, thanks to my daughter, I learned also about Timothy O'Neill's Tom Bombadil and Goldberry.   It so happened that this learning (acquisition of knowledge) coincided with the kind of life-changing experience so well described by Peter Ouspensky and, then, J.B. Priestley.

Because these things fitted so perfectly with the Jung-Plato paradigm, I perceived, professionally, that a massive weight of evidence was being accumulating in favour of that proposition.   However, the conclusive phenomena for me were two experiential occasions that were far more significant (emotionally and statistically) than *any* alternative explanation.

The two occasions to which I refer contained information that was so precise and so unique that, I believe, they could *only* have been accessed from the mind-set of an 'Other' to whose brain/mind I was 'tuned', and to whom I was emotionally close.   Since then, the notion of an elective or eclectic Platonic affinity being one's Animus/ Anima' and one's psychagogue has grown ever stronger.

(xii) The Foe

We have, therefore, to consider the impediments to not only affinitive search, but also to the class or category of impediments to all relationships in our world of relationships and fields.   I will not dignify such opposition to progress by terms such as 'enemy' or 'foe' but will call it (after Jung) 'Evil as determinant reality' that is to be fought, within the physical universe akin to a 'battlefield far and wide' (Sherrington).

Our opposition in the conflict is composed of three elements or functionaries that are dominated, widely and opportunistically, by one entity perceived (re the modern world) by Ludwig von Bertalanffy as 'the social Leviathan) and illustrated (and exemplified) brilliantly by C.S. Lewis, in *That Hideous Strength* and *The Screwtape Letters*.

In tune with my emphasis over the last few pages on classical themes, I should mention the work by Charles Seltman entitled, *The Twelve Olympians*.   In my context, he makes two significant contributions to the argument.   First, Seltman gives a splendid 31-line description of Penelope's dawning and joyous acceptance of Odysseus's identity, to which I referred earlier (pp. 93-4).

Second, he offers six ways in which modern society has need of input from those early pagan Greeks.   It is noteworthy that they placed much more value on the institution of familial marriage than they did about its 'shackling' of Love (pp. 188-9).

Charles Seltman listed, in particular, First, a zeal for Truth, Second, Humility *in the Church*,   Third, the abandonment of active *proselytism*.   Fourth, less emphasis on sin and more on 'folly'.   Fifth, more trust in the frequent *good intentions* of mankind (which do sometimes get implanted).   Sixth, Toleration – and honest toleration – must abound.

However, the aptness of the warship analogy – from, say, neurophysiology to the ancient Greeks – solicits an *ontological imperative*.   This is, perhaps illustrated best by a conversion from the saying of a Christian saint (and an attitude belonging to Omar Khayyam) to one that is shorter and more direct.   In short, it changes St. Augustine's '*Love and do what you will*' to ' Love and protect that love'.

(xiii) The Extra Requirement

Paying due respect to Dylan Thomas (and to poets and Poetry, in general, in a work that interlaces Science with it Philosophy, I must start with the thoughts of the great C.S. Sherrington upon *Man and his Nature*.   Sherrington perceived man as being immersed in a colossal battle in which his foes were Nature, Man, and Man himself.   Nature's aim for Man was to Love passionately wherever love can be felt.   *Altuism as Passion*.

The next step might be more specific but it is more conjectural (or so it can be argued).   I refer to Rollo May's ontological assertion that is certainly appropriate to Sherrington's.   [So we move from neurophysiology to psychiatry.]   In *Love and Will* Rollo May describes what happens in human experience is the succession: 'I conceive-I can-I will-I am'.   And, after having pointed out on the same page (p. 243) the element of will in Intentionality.

Elsewhere in his splendid (and necessary) book May asserts that Man's purpose is to unite Love and Will.   Although he does not list Sherington in his Index, and I don't remember redinh his name, it is clear the Sherrington and May are sending the same message from their respective standpoints. Therefore, I take the bold step of proposing the sequence, in our material world of relationships, a merger of their sayings.

I am satisfied that man's cognition is sufficient for us to dispense with the element 'I am' and, so , I replace it with something akin to 'I Love', 'I must *protect*'. Perhaps the Jesuits would prefer the term 'I must protect and nurture' – I would not object (provided they could eschew undue active proselytism).

[Personally, I would include *another* term, i.e. 'I must fight', and I realize that this is likely to offend very many people, but it is the truth and it match's the milieu described by Sherrington.] Talking of which brings me to Jung's contribution to the picture being painted. His contribution, per se, is the consolidation of the term 'must' into a categorical imperative.

This is because he asserted that Evil is *determinant reality*. There is nothing particularly earth-moving about this – it is almost a truism, and it certainly squares with Sherrington. The feature that raises Jung's status so much (to such a level that it ranks, in my opinion, with Plato) arose inadvertently.

He produced a remarkable description of the attributes and functions of *Personality* but ascribed it to his notion of a non-material *psyche*. It is only when this description is found to apply to a real-time computer system that its true value becomes apparent. Jung was *au fait* with particle physics (of his time), but was (in my opinion) inclined to err on matters metaphysical.

I can express this quite simply (but loosely) in terms of systems. In those terms (see von Bertalanffy) he was excellent on Systems Theory and on Systems Technology, but weak on Systems Philosophy. His failings were specifically (and conspicuously) in Purpose and Motivation, but the encephalization of Mind and Ego-Awareness more than redeems all that. The 'redemption' is so complete that from now on I will concentrate on matters falling into the Realm of the 'Jung-Plato paradigm'

(xiv) Jung's Contributions

In this section I speak in terms of Jungian theory being 'Revisited' by me. The degree of 'Refreshment' is for my readers to decide. This follows on logically from the previous section, wherein I *correct* Jung's ideas on Purpose and Motivation. I make no bones about it – there is little place in a world of relationships and fields for Jungian Individualism.

In fact, there is not much to change. Jung spoke of *cosmogonic love* and was extremely drawn to the notion of 'elective affinities'; and Plato wrote of 'affinitive search' among many 'lookalikes'. There may be a slight difference between them in that Plato spoke of a 'Charioteer' disciplining his highly unruly black horse, whereas Jung espoused 'responsibility' rather than 'self-control'.

Both, however, saw Reincarnation as being the vehicle of their 'doom' – one way or another. And, both were equally harsh. Plato conceived of *metempsychosis* [which is a 'scary' notion] while Jung perceived a 'Creative Determinant' visiting upon us 'the sins we have thought, intended, or committed' [equally scary, but less likely].

More likely than either of these possibilities, however, is the scenario afforded by the systems approach (because it is based upon models). From a systems viewpoint, consonant with Whitehead's process philosophy, an equally daunting prospect awaits a person who is not, so to speak, 'up to scratch' or 'up to it'.

A systems model, under those conditions, would have the ultimate user – for whom the system or process was designed – able to obliterate the 'process image' or to suspend temporarily its implementations. Nobody else can do this except, possibly, the 'systems engineer'. If THE USER did decide to do either, then the implemented process might become one of Jung's 'detached' processes or, in more dramatic terms a 'zombie'.

Jung has a vital role in our comprehension of (a) the phenomena of _Mystical Indwelling_ and (b) _our Experiencing of Level_. At its face value the statement may be surprising, but the role was an _enabling_ one. It enables us to understand how the analogies of a lift in a lift-shaft and of water in a well can be consistent with each other – they refer to different phenomena. And, moreover, they apply to _real_ phenomena.

This is not the case with the beliefs held on Love at the Sapientic level, which is now open to discussion in a new paradigm. The same attributes and functions hold after three millennia but, from being attributes of the Gods, they are now to be seen as properties of, in order, the Brain/ Mind(Ego), the 'Soul-body', and the Spirit-body'.

For example, William Johnston's 'progression' of Love to the stage of Sapientia is parallel to the consequences Eros's 'arrow' striking its target. In the case of sexual union being accompanied by Love, the act (called 'aphrodite' by Greeks) takes the loving relationship into the province of Eros's mother, namely the goddess 'Aphrodite'.

Upon this happening, her sister goddesses, Hera (marriage), Athene (Learning) and Hestia (Hearth), rapidly converge, and the four goddesses make a very strong call for the consideration of Zeus (and possibly Ares?). An impressive description and commentary is given by Charles Seltman in _The Twelve Olympians_ (pp, 78-9).

A key feature, fastened upon by many and interpreted correctly by few, is Jung's quaternion of _attitudes_, namely Eve, Helen, Mary, and Sapientia. Although his choice of examples may seem weird, his underlying notion, of _growth_, is brilliant. The ascension describes the _expansion_ of one's emotional compass or range, within the physical universe in accordance with increases in our learning and knowledge and experience.

The increase, for Jung, was always seen to result from the pursuit of an 'Anticipated Whole Other', which for Jung was a construct entirely fictive, stochastic, and disposable. For everybody else, the 'Anticipated Whole Other' is real and it relates to one's _soul-mate_ (as in Plato). One can appreciate this best through the Sino-Asiatic model.

In this model, Soul-Mates are separate physical entities throughout the physical universe, but the forces that drive the material bodies towards each other in the physical universe, cooperate with each other within a _higher level system_, outside the physical universe. This is what Jung could not, or would not, concede (except by reference to 'cosmogonic love' as God).

This concept *is* extremely difficult to grasp, and few relationships reach this level (as Jung pointed out in terms of individuals). William Johnston understands and explains it for us very well in terms of the expansion through the 'quaternic ascension' and into mystical union, merger, and indwelling (and the associated gathering of learning and knowledge).

The point he makes extremely well is that much of the functionality is concomitant and stretches from the level of 'Simultaneity' down to that of 'Instantaneity' through 'passing time' – a triage that is modelled both in mathematics and in real-time computer systems. In other words, these notions are existential *and* experiential.

Jung's differentiation between *Intuition* and *Feeling* leads us to an appreciation and understanding of *mystical indwelling* that supports William Johnston in ways scientific and, yet, experiential. Ways not open to laboratory testing and control, but in touch with the man/woman in the street – just as Priestley found out with his 'mass observation' through TV.

Another 'mass observation' lends support to this claim – that of Scott Williamson and Innes Pearse (both medical doctors) - in a long-running experiment in community health, the benefits of which were measured in terms of overall health and well-being. The 'Peckham Experiment', as it was called, lasted between the years 1926 -1951 and it yielded significantly positive results.

(xv) The Peckham Experiment

I mention Williamson and Pearse chiefly because their experiment was geared to measurement over a long period of time and a not unreasonable 'sample size' obtaining in 'normal' everyday life. Their work has a few other features that are worthy of brief mention, but to understand it and to convey meaning is difficult because one has to learn and understand a whole new language to do so.

Nevertheless, nearly half the pages in *Science, Synthesis and Sanity* have interesting reliance for me in the context of my argument, so I feel that another few paragraphs won't be misspent. For example, the first page that I have just opened at random contains the sentences: 'It is as though the mutual attraction which we see in sex were applied to the synthesis of all apposite specific diversities. They come together by some mutual qualificatory attraction' (p. 57).

These two sentences appear to cover eventualities from, say, 'elective affinities' to Mattessich's 'systems principles' especially when the very next sentence include the simile of locks fitting keys within a 'field of familiarity', and the text being within a subsection headed *Eclectivity*. [the concept of locks fitting keys is an interesting one]

Another interesting concept is the use of the term 'functionary'. If we relate this to mechanistic embodiment, then the term seems to apply to the Determinator rather than the Agent – although both come under it. We have the statement that: 'Function is concerned not with *what* is done but with *how* it is done' (p.35).

The relevance of that statement is, in particular, that it is included in the context of there being 'a world of confusion' about the terms 'quality' and 'quantity' (p. 36). The text goes on to accentuate the *very serious difficulty that quality cannot be defined or measured in any positive fashion,...,* but at the time of writing I.J. Good's subjective probability was just in its early infancy.

In fact, to all intents and purpoes, the closure of the Peckham experiment coincided with the advent of real-time military computer systems. Sixty years on, the difference in status of the Agent and the Determinator as functionaries has diminished greatly, as the former has gained an enormous amount of autonomy and the latter has declined in terms of Command.

We can understand more easily today that the Agent and the Determinator determine *how* their respective functions are to operate in fields *at different levels.* The former has considerable license in generating maximal operational efficiency, and the latter has equal freedom in ensuring mission completion. *Always*, of course, within the parameters laid down for each in the Specification that is an *Ideal Form.*

It is notable that *autonomy* and *action-pattern,* and *Memory-Will and Aesthesia,* and *Potential for Action*, and many other apparently apposite terms are given attention in the large 'Dictionary of Quality' which occupies thirty pages towards the end of *Science, Synthesis and Sanity.*

Our concentration may be focussed upon the contents of pages 256 and 258, in which it is written (compositely) that the aim of the authors is to help the recognition of 'mind' being something distinctly different from 'psyche', and both as different from the 'functionary'. Also, that 'soul' might reasonably be equated with the functionary; and, in that context, 'soul is a property of all organism'.

In another sense, soul might be reasonably equated with the 'artist, poet, mystic, theologian, and the scientist', and might well find a future meeting place, i.e. in their location in the dimension of Memory-Will. This, they say, is not the soul or psyche of the psychologist, nor of any other technologist, but the simpler soul of our forefathers.

In their complete honesty, Williamson and Pearse remark that neither Memory-Will nor the presence of the functionary in that dimension tells us of the essential 'origin' of Life: any more than the dimension Space-Time of the physicist tells us of the essential source or 'origin' of Energy. These are the 'How' questions that lead to the positing of a <u>functionary</u> – symbol for the existence of a *directive* of the directable organic mechanism.

I have given Williamson and Pearse the status of a numbered section in Part Two because they *seem* so consonant with the Sino-Asiatic model of Reality, on the one hand, and with particle physics and mechanistic embodiment, on the other hand. There is much more of interest in this fascinating little book, such as 'eclectivity in will' (p. 257), which surely would have interested Rollo May, and a great deal of attention to 'Feeling', which likewise would have interested Jung. However, I feel it is time for me to return to Mysticism and Jung

(xvi) The Question of Levels

In all these matters, differences in level can be regarded as differences between major or minor realms along the Axis of Scale. And , for me, the axis of scale is immensely useful in conveying Scale as a dimension (see Rucker).   It comes in useful, also, in trying to convey the 'nesting' of systems hierarchically.

I find it very difficult to represent this kind of 'nesting' which takes place in the Sino-Asiatic model, but I always have in mind Figure E7-2 (page 360) of *The Self and Its Brain* by Popper and Eccles.   I would   like to offer the same format, i.e. a re-arranged block diagram with different meanings, but it eludes me at present.

It may be that Popper and Eccles are attempting to portray information flow within the 'strong dualistic hypothesis', while I am trying to indicate structured nesting within Comprehensive Reality.   Donald MacKay's scheme   might almost be called the construct of a physicalist, but certainly not a materialistic one.   At least, not in the sense given by Steven Rose.

It seems that the question of *level* is ever-present.   It is not mentioned explicitly by Williamson and Pearse, but it is clearly present in their text.   I believe that they made the same error in communication as did Popper and Ecccles.   I feel that this error has cost Science, Philosophy (not to mention Religion) dear.

However, *The Self and Its Brain does* give us valuable information about the brain, and *Science, Synthesis and Sanity* leaves us with not only many intriguing notions, but also knowledge of a rare kind in this field.   As I said earlier, the experiment was properly measured over a community for a long time, and, unknown to Williamson and Pearse, their ideas *can*, in principle, be awarded quantitative weightings.

The question of scale and level, in the context of Jung and Mysticism, can be approached best (in my opinion) by way of comparing notions of David Bohm's concept of individuals in their immense environment with those Realms along the axis of scale encountered in the Sino-Asiatic model – they both tie-in with particle physics and transcendental or theistic Mysticism. This, it seems to me, equates roughly with Plato's 'One and the Many'.

To do this, I have to deal with ideas with which I am unsure and aspects of mathematics that are (well) outside my capabilities, but it has to be done.   I begin, therefore, by citing Michael Talbot's *THE HOLOGRAPHIC UNIVERSE*, which I have used, until now, as an excellent 'source book' but without referring to it.   I will use it now for the consolidation of my own ideas and experience – not without some reluctance.

Therefore, I now cite David Bohm's belief that subatomic particles possess a distinct reality without consciousness entering the picture (p. 139).   Bohm also believes that every region of space is awash with different kinds of fields composed of waves of varying lengths.   This 'infinite ocean of energy', he thinks, *does* exist, and it tells us at least a little about the 'vast and hidden nature' of an 'implicate order' (p. 51).

David Bohm believes that Space is a ground for the existence of everything , including ourselves.   The universe is just a ripple on the surface of this cosmic sea of energy. It is a comparatively small 'pattern of excitation' in the midst of an 'unimaginably vast ocean', and this notion seems extremely close to my comprehension of a 'pattern of excitation' sweeping through 'mathematical Platonism'.

However, we are cautioned that this does not mean that the universe is 'a giant undifferentiated mass'. Things can be part of an undivided whole and still possess their own qualities (p. 48), and this is where I start to waver. The Realms to which I refer along the axis of scale may be separated by 'indefinite boundaries' (see Playfair), but they are separated, also, by a number of orders of magnitude – which is much more persuasive.

David Bohm's 'ripple' is the same universe as is portrayed by Lee Smolin, which consists only of relationships and fields, and has nothing outside it. In contradistinction to this, the Sino-Asiatic model has Spirit-Bodies both inside and outside the universe. In the latter case, they are levels of divinity (see Motoyama).

In the former case, however, we have the levels that accord with the sub-realms delineated by the levels of atoms, fermions, quarks, and several putative extra layers. The Spirit-Body inhabits all Realms but, in the universe, it is joined by the Soul-Body which allows the Yin and the Yang principles to manifest Women and Men, respectively.

Jung and non-transcendental Mysticism are the features obtaining in all sub-realms of this basic Realm of Physicality   And, it seems likely that all clairvoyance and extra-sensory perception are within the physical Realm.

(xvii) Sapientia and Synchronicity

In similar vein to the preceding text, this subject has been given the status of a numbered section because of its use by Jung, and/or the Jungians of his time, and because of its appositeness to my *experience*, which I offer as *evidence*, The Jungian notion of 'Sapientia' is a fictive, concocted and disposable construct. In rather stark contrast, my notion of Sapientia (from my experience) is real, experiential, and relational.

In fact, my definition of the state of Sapientia , *ad hoc*, might be: a state of *Permanent, Ineffable, One-ness, Undemanding*, and *Selfless*, i.e, 'PIOUS'. The acronym pleases me, but it should not be taken as an indication of any kind of religious belief for three reasons, at least. First, my adherence to scientific principles prohibits religion, other than Natural Theology. Second, it is indicative of a *relationship* but the term refers to individual poles of the relationship. Third, it relates to a *Feeling* of 'uplift'.

The *Shorter Oxford English Dictionary* is the only dictionary among a dozen or so in my personal library which includes Sapientia. It gives: 'Sapientia -   Wisdom, Understanding, Correct Taste or Judgment'. Likewise, that Dictionary gives one (rare) definition of Pious as being 'faithful to the natural requirements of loving relationships' This is what I meant by the term, and it is consonant with my other remarks. However, in terms of *Mysticism*, William Johnston gives a reference that requires my comment.

He describes a 'growth' from the erotic to the mystical in relation to Love, and my first comment is only to suggest that 'expansion' might be a preferable term (p. 139 of *The*

Inner Eye of Love).   My second comment, however, is of more consequence – it pertains to Jung's well-known hierarchy of Eve, Helen of Troy, the Virgin Mary, and Sapientia or Wisdom.   I make no comment about the choice of characters, but continue with my attention to Mysticism (and mystical union, merger, and indwelling).

Johnston ascribes to Jung the idea that 'human love should grow and develop through these stages', and my second comment is that Jung affirmed and re-affirmed that 'the goal of psychic development is the self' - and the Jungian 'problematic', even today, is the distinction between 'Self' and 'Other'.   William Johnston, moreover, avers that an 'affinitive' relationship produces both the highest personalism _and_ the highest union.

In *Man and his Symbols*, it is made quite clear that, to a Jungian, Sapientia is the final stage of the growth of the *Anima/ Animus*, which develops up to the level of a construct called 'the Anticipated Whole Other' and is then disposed of because the goal of psychic development, the self, has been reached.

Unless William Johnston had other and better knowledge of Jung, this popular misconception remained until Timothy O'Neill restored the integrity of Jungian theory by presenting the proper identification of the Yin and Yang principles from which Jung and/or his followers (at the time) departed.

It is noteworthy that Sapientia pertains to the individual.   For example, the interpretation of Jungian theory by William Johnston is in terms of *individuals* reaching that state and _then_ uniting, or merging, or indwelling.   William Johnston's highest level is whereat individuals join with divinity.

We owe it to Peter Ouspensky that, by the *tertium organum*, i.e. intuitive logic, we are taken into some 'higher' level in the physical universe at which *relationships* are at the point of reaching divinity but have various karmas – individual and shared – to release before proceding along their chosen path.   Through Ouspensky we can talks in such terms that we understand Jung and the Sino-Asiatic model (see Motoyama).

All of any discussion centres upon the crux of the Jungian problematic, i.e. that the Jungian modes of Perception and Judgment – the four functions – are or *are no*t in relation to Others.   For Jungians they were completely self-referential and, for some, they still are.

The only interest such Jungians have in the Other is in how (in their perception and judgment) 'the Other' (past, present, and future) might affect the journey to the Self. This Self-absorption leads to justifiable caustic comments, such as those made by Anthony Storr, and surely that position can no longer be maintained..

It follows from this that the various mechanisms supposed to be supportive of ESP (*Extra-Sensory Perception*) are still open to our investigations.   As John Polkinghorne remarks, it is reasonable to suppose that if they affect the material world, we should be able to discern them.   However, almost by definition, it does not follow that we should be able to measure them [although we can assess quantitatively their Likelihood].

This leads me to the question of *Evidence*, and I affirm, freely and willingly, that I have experienced the phenomena of Clairvoyance on a dozen or so occasions.   I cover most of the instances (scientifically recorded as soon as possible after the event) in the Appendix, and I must record here that the style and the content (but _not_ their interpretation) are very similar to Jung's 'visions' and 'personifications' as he recounts them in *Memories, Dreams, Reflections*.

Speaking professionally, i.e. as an applied statistician, a good number of them imply some 'hidden' mechanism and could not have happened by chance. Each of the dozen occasions featured some event or mechanism as a 'kernel' of which I was unaware at the time. So, I affirm that I have experienced, on at least two occasions, the transfer from another mind to my own such knowledge of an event which I could not have gained in any other way according to the statistical laws of Likelihood. In short, I could not have *imagined* the two events.

Additionally, I have communicated with visions or personifications (in the Jungian sense) in both natural language and highly compressed data, and also via sensation. These occasions are all recorded faithfully, i.e. written down as soon as possible after the event, and they are presented in the Appendix A. [I have also communicated (apparently) with a small bird]

Each vision (including Personifications) comes to us by courtesy of the physiological mechanisms outlined by Donald MacKay. Their details (colours, sounds, movements, moods, impressions, values, shapes, sizes, etc., etc.) are fashioned by our 'mind-sets'. And, a feature of the Jung-Plato paradigm is that the mind-sets, per se, may be influenced by a psychagogue and/or Animus/ Anima.

Be that as it may, if we assume that all the affects and influences of this kind of 'lay' mysticism take place within the physical universe, then it has been found useful by many to perceive Stratification within the universe. Each field of thought seems to have its own 'version' of this conception – and Jungian theory is no exception to this.

As I have just indicated, Sapientia is at the highest level or stratum in a hierarchy of at least four levels. William Johnston chooses to associate this with the development of mystical love, and this squares with Livesey's concept of emotion developing with learning and with MacKay's mechanistic embodiment.

The notion also ties-in with Aristotle's notions of increasing system complexity, and with Whitehead's construct of *Togetherness* as a universal aim and need, and, too, with Sherrington's idea of the development of 'Altruism as Passion'. Jung will not be left out of this, because of his hierarchy of collectivity and its networks of communication at each level.

And, with the networks come higher centres of Command and Communications *and* the relational knowledge-bases and the various methods of *chaining* together isolated pieces of information upon which intercommunication between and within levels can take place.

In Part Three, I give a kind of 'expanded Glossary' which serves, also, to afford some indication, at least, of how 'trains of thought', 'flows of consciousness', hypnagogic imagery, visions and personifications, Sapientic telepathy and so on, can be imagined and, perhaps, even modelled.   I shall touch again on this 'mechanization' in this current Part Two and Part Three.

Synchronicity, therefore, does not contain the significance attributed to it by many authors – it is merely the consequence of chains of networks and relational storage. However, these _factual_ processes _should_ add to the authority and the   power of psycholinguistic analysis (see the Appendix).   Animal reaction symbols should be advanced considerably by the notion (and humans too).

In short, whatever may lie outside the physical universe, its stratification is not only earmarked for us by particle physics, any demarcation is also furnished by the 'limits' and 'bounds' provided by Science and by the philosophies of the East and Middle East, I,e, the Sino-Asiatic model.

(xviii) The Universe of Symbols and Man's Quaternic Environment

Musing, when Dawn's left hand was in the sky (_pace_ Fitzgerald), my thoughts went to the works of the founder of General Systems Theory, Ludwig von Bertalanffy (_pace_ Aristotle).   I was thinking, particularly, of his theory of _Perspectivism_.

I reflected that this was almost a truism, and that it could be used as a _quaternion_ in the Jungian sense.   Four elements can be discerned in Man's conflict with the social Leviathan (and other evils).   The one that is different from the others is Symbols, created by Mankind (!?) and perceived by him/her.   The others (loosely) are Images (generated by the brain (see MacKay)) and/or, more generally, by Action Systems (applicable to all cellular organisms), and 'Action Information Systems' (likewise).

Reflecting further, I thought of my acronym, PIOUS, in terms of perspectives and realized that many other personalities or identities could be be formed from it , not only for myself but also for categorizing others.   For example, the letter 'I' could represent, say, not only 'Ineffable' but also   'Inaccessible', 'Intimate', 'Informed', 'Irreligious', 'Invigorate', 'Inspirational', Illuminating', 'Illustrious', 'irrepressible' etc., not all of which have direct opposites.

Clearly, this might be a useful and searching analytical tool,   However, my purpose, here, is to lead into a final, detailed, depiction of the Jungian characteristics of what has become known as an 'Intelligent Support System'.   But, before this, I must re-iterate that brain/mind(Ego) appear to be, beyond doubt, the product of Biological Evolution.

This distinguishing between 'function' and 'functionary' is not just theoretical.   It comes, we surmise, from the 'triune brain' which, itself, is part of an 'embodied formula' that corresponds to a wave of activity sweeping through mathematical Platonism (according to the Jung-Plato paradigm).   Not so for Jung.   Jung states that 'Man is _raised out of_ the animal world' by virtue of his reflective faculties' (p. 312).

(xix) An Intelligent Support System

(a) General

Continuing with this kind of theme of embodiment, one often encounters the variety of thoughts provided by William James. It is not altogether surprising that Jung makes very little reference to him, but there *are* aspects and perspectives which could have been mentioned, such as the *superconscious,* and the *stream of consciousness,* and *polytheism and plurality,* which would have been of interest and not too discordant with Jung's ideas.

However, we can set aside, in this section, Jung's notions of transcendental, monotheistic, mysticism, and concentrate upon the 'lay' mysticism of William James in regard of mystical transfer of information and knowledge. That is to say, we focus upon Individuals in the Jumgian state of Sapientia – just before or below the transcendental levels of divinity.

I must mention, at this point, that the philosophy of William James was nominated as *Neutral Monism,* and it is not discordant with Perspectivism, Mechanistic Embodiment, Particle Physics, Cosmology, and Whitehead's Process Philosophy, but it does conflict with Donald MacKay's belief that no 'etherial' representation of an Ideal Form is necessary.

The philosophy of William James is *very* consonant with our present concept of such a placement of Ideal Forms within the physical universe. Indeed, it consolidates our suspicions that only two kinds of Ideal Form exist. The first is that in the physical universe they can only be conceptual and 'perfect' in the mind's eye. The second kind is the notion of a *specification* of prescription and proscription.

Returning to the Jamesian analysis of (lay) mystical experience, the two <u>significant</u> occasions to which I referred earlier (re my Acronym of PIOUS) were characterized by their *Transience,* and William James had transience as one of his characteristics of mystical insight featuring in (pages thirty-four to thirty-six) of Johnston's text on mystical knowledge in his *The Inner Eye of Love.*

Another characteristic feature is that of *Ineffability* which, he writes 'James, very simply and very wisely, attributes this ineffability to the fact that mystical states are more like states of <u>feeling</u> (my emphasis) than states of intellect'.

A third characteristic is that of *noetic quality* giving <u>real knowledge</u> that is illuminative, revelatory, and significant. The cognitive content of mystical knowledge is non-conceptual and belongs to a different state of consciousness. Hence, great caution must be used in reporting it.

Yet another feature is that the transience of the occasion masks an underlying <u>permanent state</u> (my emphasis), a deep peace that is compatible with many experiences – good or bad. All this is most undramatic, says William Johnston, but it is truly mystical; it is the work of love in those deeper [higher?] levels of consciousness.

He goes on to refer to other features at other levels, but I think I have done enough to indicate a considerable overlap of my three significant experiences with standard features of mystical experience just below the level of divinity.

There is more, much more, in this book, but I cannot move on without citing a page (p. 155) which – as I typed – fell open to reveal a line which I had previously underlined: 'Discernment is the essence of mysticism in action'(!).   [Which seems particularly appropriate.]

William Johnston's pages on mystical knowledge are founded upon those of William James, before him.   In truth, the vast contribution made by James could be measured by the number of people citing him or quoting him.   I can join that countless number by pointing out (and 'modelling') two particular features of his wide-spread talent.

The first of these refers to his notion of a 'stream of consciousness'.   This corresponds, quite closely, to the sequential flow of processing in a real-time computer.   I mention elsewhere in this book how, at base, the computer breaks down sequentially the operations and locations in each   *word* of a computer program to produce a 'flow' of conversion from *potential* to *actual*.

But, here, I am referring to the succession through the 'plurality of consciousness' as the 'flow of conversion' passes through a dozen or more *'nested interrupts'* .   I have actually represent this process diagrammatically in a technical memorandum, as I have also represented the frequency at which different functions are performed, (see Figure 3 for both).

I can't remember cross-correlating these with the biorhythms illustrated in *Silent Music: The Science of Meditation*, but my intention throughout much of my working life was to attach measuring devices to a computer's operating system so as to generate *its* 'biorhythms. [I never got round to it].

The other feature, to which I referred, is the citation, made by Ludwig von Bertalanffy in *Robots, Men and Minds*, of the Jamesian description of how an organism creates (in a very real sense) the world about it.   In regard of this, we know today that the organism does this along the course of evolution – from protozoa to humans.

In fact, von Bertalanffy *does* refer to 'innumerable factors arising in biological evolution' (p. 91) and to the 'active, psychophysical organism' having not only motoric or 'output' behaviour but also 'input' to cognitive processes (p. 92).

In 1967, therefore, we find the nucleus of future distinctions between function and functionary, agent and determinator, extraversion and introversion, etc., and subsequent sections on 'the Mind-Body Problem' and, then, ' Unitary Theory'.   Whereas, *General System Theory* sets out much on the principles of organisms as 'Action Systems', *Robots, Men and Minds* discusses 'psychology in the modern World', and both books are still are invaluable to students some fifty years on.

However, in this subsection, I wish to draw attention to the words of L. von Bertalanffy on William James in which he writes: '...in a very real sense, the organism *creates* the world around it.   William James' "buzzing, 'blooming', confusion" of sense data is molded, as it were, by human categories If we speak in philosophical language; in terms of Psychology, by innumerable factors arising in biological evolution' (1967, p. 91).

Splendid examples of this – also of Jung's hypnagogic imagery – are to be found in the dimly-lit *operations rooms* of operational warships with their profusion of flickering and ever-changing images on VDU (Visual Display Unit) screens, each dealing with a different area of attention.   If we replace the human element, as with MacKay's Comprehensiv Reality, then the sense of 'buzzing, blooming, confusion' becomes very much enhanced.   But, it can be recorded and analysed.

Exactly the same considerations apply to the mechanization of mind-like processes in the hierarchies of Command, Control and Communication obtaining not only in military circles but gradually creeping into Commerce and Politics as limbs of the social Leviathan.

For example, 'relational' knowledge bases and data bases use redundancy of information to gain time at the expense of storage, or 'data- chaining' to save storage at the cost of speed.   'Special' memories record vital information for reconfiguring after damage or breakdown and the 'operations' room is separate from the 'bridge' in a warship, and is more heavily protected, for similar reasons

Much information is held, also, in regard of what might be classified as 'social', even in military systems, and I will expand on this in the following subsection.   Finally, therefore, I leave my readers with a rhetorical question which could provide amusement at the right kind of dinner-party.

William James, himself , pointed out that essential and fundamental discernment in human thought lies in the distinction between the issues of *'Me'* and *'Not-Me'*.   This was in 1890 (Ornstein Ed., 1973, p. 166), so our rhetorical question(s) is 'What would he have thought of Ouspensky/ Priestley/ Bennett?'   Or of C.G. Jung?   Or Sherrington?   Or Motoyama?

(b) Detail

(i) On Nomenclature

I use the term 'Action System' because it is comparatively free of 'theory loading' and it suits my purpose of covering the process of Evolution from protozoa to the most highly developed human brain.   The term was coined by David Clarke (with Jill Crosland) as an introduction to complex behaviour which studies and unifies 'natural behaviour in all its complexity'.

The protozoan has every right to be included under such a heading, in some way it manages to seek escape from predators, seek nutrients, reproduce its kind (by sexual and/or asexual reproduction), survive hostile environments (encyst), move to more 'healthy' surroundings, etc., all according to its 'inner state'.   It even (apparently) seeks company.

There must be, in the terms of Donald MacKay, *some* kind of 'determinator', because the system works.   The actions are determined – the little creature survives.   Its walk is not random, and Roger Penrose believes that, in some way(s), it reaches outside space and time in communication with others.   This is cold, calm, proper, scientific conjecture which joins with similar conjectures from other eminently respectable scientists.

(ii) The Relocation of Personality

By this, I mean the re-attribution of every detail of 'Personality', which Jung attributed to a non-material 'psyche', to a material, functioning brain. Hence, the term – for convenience – 'Brain/ Mind(Ego)'. This, now, covers *all* features given by Jung to personality, and it *corrects* some of them. I make no apologies for this piece of seeming didacticism – the faults have been indicated by Jung's fellows.

I will particularize. Under the aegis of the Jung-Plato paradigm, the Shadow function is improved and exemplified, as is the Persona. Purpose is clarified unambiguously and is assigned to the whole 'vessel' under a Determinator function that has specialist areas concerning 'warfare', 'navigation', 'pilotage', and a Command status that is transferable according to a variety of contingencies.

Furthermore, inconsistencies in Jungian theory are 'ironed out', a prime example of which is the *re-alignment* of the four functions. Instead of Jung's pairings, Sensation is now paired with Thinking, and Intuition with Feeling. David Cox, in *Analytical Psychology* (pp. 101-9) covers the situation prior to the revamp. Anthony Stor, in *Jung*, also explains Jung's predicament (pp. 74-5).

Moreover, Emotion – assiduously excluded by Jung – is seen to permeate the whole organization (Action System) and to become a 'universal'. For example, in a civilized country, its military officers take an oath of pursuing their duty of safeguarding and nurturing Others at the cost of their life, if necessary. That dedication and fervour permeates whatever vessel they command – and each and every member of its crew.

(iii) the Shadow

The relocation of the Personality from the psyche to the evolved, material brain actually *improves* our conceptualization of the *Shadow* function. The *Purpose*, which embraces the whole Action System (aka 'vessel', 'organism', 'entity', 'whatever'), and which should reflect the Command's orientation and Mission, swims into sharp focus.

The System's 'ISS' (Intelligent Support System) possesses a compendium of checklists and Security precautions that is not only 'mind-boggling', but mind-boggling 'specific'. *Everything is* there which could conceivably damage the vessel, the Mission, an itinerary, subsidiary aims, operational performance, etc. Indeed, a military vehicle provides a prime example of how even a metaphysical assertion could easily – and seriously – affect *Behaviour*.

Examples abound. Relocation ensures that increased attention is directed towards the Other. This clerly influences Personality in numerous ways, many of which I will touch upon in this subsection. For example, the Persona – coupled with EW (Electronic Warfare) – is exemplified. Electronic Warfare (EW) and ECM (Electronic

CounterMeasures), ECCW, etc., are such *sensitive areas*, however,that I will say no more – I have signed the Official Secrets Act.

It is a point worth making that a military vessel is compelled to bring Others into consideration because it would not wish to accidentally inflict upon Others things that are undesirable for itself. For example, it would not wish to have 'foreign' aircraft flying too close to its powerful radars or have 'friendly' vessels to be demolished by its missiles.

So-called 'friendly fire' is a commonplace mishap that occurs surprisingly frequently on the small scale – and sometimes it reflects badly on the training and ethos of its perpetrators. However, on the large scale, it could be disastrous in a number of ways. For example, if a missile were to destroy a vessel belonging to a 'friendly' nation.

Except, that is, if it were to be a deliberate 'accident'.   I am being perfectly serious; and such a topic, in public airing, indicates the parlous situation in international politics today. In this arena, I am quite sure that the truth beggars imagination. Having signed the Official Secrets Act (in 1948), I am still acutely conscious of of being told of some things that I must *never, ever* mention them to *anyone*.

These are just some of the ways in which the vessel is *forced* to communicate with Others – the mundane, material world is so vastly different from Jung's world of a hypothesized psychical 'mind(Ego)'. [It makes one wonder how such a conjectured entity could ever be expected to work in the material domain]

It follows that, in psychological terms, Ruth Munroe's (Freudian) wording seems quite adequate for describing Jung's 'collective unconscious'. That is to say: it is 'a set of universals, operative and becoming manifest, at the bio-social level'. Or, in the words of A.N. Whitehead, it is simply 'an organized set of subjective aims'.

Such things I have felt and observed from experience. For example, a collective of warships makes an excellent example – it s a collective of 'hybrid' action systems that is open to classification in a number of ways. In a single vessel, there is a 'Gestalt' formed by a blending of emotions towards a common purpose.

This, within a single vessel, is enhanced and magnified – encouraged and fostered by the Command – into feelings of solidarity, camaraderie, singularity of Mission, exultation (and sometimes grief), etc., into a considerable force. Often myths and legends are used (and sometimes created), but they are only tools.

An example, from my own experience, is the 'corporate grief' that swept throughout the Portsmouth area when H.M.S. Hood was sunk during WW2 – it was almost palpable. The words, 'The Hood's gone down', seemed to echo throughout the region, and then a kind of doom-laden hush descended. Later, the announcement of Victory precipitated 'corporate joy'.

As it happens, I became a rifleman, in the King's Royal Rifle Corps, immediately after the cessation of hostilities, and I experienced the same kind of feeling. I still do so – some seven decades later!   The *right kind* of genuine elites of quality is of enormous benefit to a society and its causes, and we see this daily on 'newscasts'.

I _must_ repeat – out of respect for J.B. Priestley and other veterans and heroes of the war – that my military service started just after the war ended. However, this does not signify that I did not experience terror during 'blitzes' during the war. And, during my service in the 60th Rifles, I witnessed the roughest and toughest of men benefitting, as I was, from the development of 'esprit de corps' and discipline.

None of this pertains to any kind of 'mythopoeic imagination' as Jung asserted. It belongs, fairly and squarely, to our brains and the considerable number of 'situation generators', 'character generators', 'symbols generators', 'scenario generatos', etc., that they possess. And, it happens in the ways shown so admirably by Donald MacKay and Ernest Kent.

(iv) The Persona

Whereas the Shadow is self-orientated, the Persona is more 'Other-orientated', in the sense that we are still hiding the truth about ourselves behind a mask. The two functions overlap; but they have in common that they adapt according to their Mission Objective. Perhaps we could say that the Shadow hides things away, or 'buries' them, and the Persona makes things look different.

It is unfortunate that ths savours of deceit, but that's life. There are people who never tell even 'white' lies, but I wouldn't want be be one of them. Apart from 'fibbing' to spare feelings, it is natural to want to show oneself in the best light. There are people who go too far in this, but, again, I would not want to be one of them. [Groucho Marx comes to mind]

This is, generally, applicable to an action system; but it is particularly appropriate to a warship. Its Persona might be described as: 'The attitude taken to convey special meaning to, or to hide meaning from, others…in essence, a _necessity_ for encounters with others, particularly in regard of Mission requirements…the demeanours corresponding to the needs of the Mission, in particular, and of operational life, in general'. [I can't remember the origins of this definition; it may even have been saved from old papers of my own – it fits anyway].

There are many striking parallels or analogies between warship and human, and, at times, the former can seem just like an extension of the latter's body. Most of the ship's 'Persona' patterns of behaviour have to do with the formalities of protocols, 'understandings', relationships, intentions, and so on, involved with international politics between great powers or authorities. However, at the lower end of the scale, the Persona can be of critical importance.

'Gunboat Diplomacy', for example, is still practiced, although it is gradually giving way to other forms of coercion or extortion – other weapons have taken over from guns. In terms of international tension 'airspace' is a very sensitive issue. Even in times of little tension, it is highly advisable for any kind of vessel rapidly approaching the vicinity of a capital warship to make absolutely clear its identity and intentions.

In more peaceful times, say in ceremonial affairs, crew members will line the decks of a warship on entering or leaving harbour – failure to do so might be taken 'wrongly'. Likewise, displays of bunting on special occasions.   Protocols of this type are too numerous to list; and on some occasions, their absence, or the way they are carried out, may give offence (and, be meant to do so).

However, the Persona has appositive and constructive side to it that is common to human and to warship.   Emotions may have to be masked, and grief, anxiety, apprehension, dubiety, etc., may need to be hidden.   All these things come under leadership and initiative; and, even with modern computers, may usually be entrusted to the man/woman in command.

(v) Defence Mechanisms and (vi) Trickery and Guile

These two items are so close to human nature that – wishing to preserve a smooth flow of narrative – I can only identify them here and expand upon them in later items {nos. (xvi) and (xvii)}.   There are other considerations, such as Security and my own Personal Involvement (research –wise).

However, I _can_ point out here the insufficiency of Jung's notions of Archetypes in terms of Individuals.   This is alredy wide-spread and it is ever-spreading.   It thrusts itself upon our attention and there is (seemingly) no obvious way of dealing with it.   I refer, of course, to the proliferation of 'scams' and 'abuses' that divides human beings into 'fools' and 'knaves'.

Each trickster of abuser has (usually) a number of 'gullibles', and _vice versa_, and this lends itself or 'demands' the categorical acceptance, in a world of relationships, of such a distinction between relational types.   In my opinion, the classification of a person, thus, should be a formal part of personality assessment.

(vi)   Time Dimensions

Covered in Part Three.

(vii) Linguistic Analysis and Semiotics

One thing leads to another, and I come now to the place of Semiotics in the evolutionary picture, and it cannot be surprising that linguistic analysis and semiotics play an important role in the military field as they do in ordinary psychological practice.

Freud and Jung initiated human activities in this direction for analysis, but C.S. Pierce formalized the structural foundations to very good effect (see Elizabeth Bates). And, the encephalization of the Mind(Ego) brings the two psychologists together into the evolutionary picture.

I will cite merely two particular Jungian contributions.   First, is Jung's development of word association tests.   Second, is his introduction of the term 'complex' for a 'cluster of emotionally toned ideas', the significance of which having been indicated already by Freud (Munroe, p. 40).

Other related techniques and approaches include such things as Free Association, Analysis of Dreams, Repertory Grids, Personal Construct Theory, Transactional Analysis, and various other scales and levels such as the Myers-Briggs set of Personality characteristics, which now requires changes and additions.

In relation to my central theme of the 'Jung-Plato paradigm', the concept of Evolution takes on a completely different, and more simple, form, to which I refer sometimes as 'a hand brushing an abacus'. Evolution is obviously on a much larger scale, but in principle it is a similar mechanism, and questions arise about the mechanism of MacKay's notion of the 'Determinator function'.

I can write only of techniques and methods that I have used myself in this field; and these pertain either to Heuristic Learning from Signs and to the analysis of its User by a software system (see Appendix). I am taking care not to claim that I have *introduced* any novel or original notions, because others may have preceded me, but I have been told so in a number of cases.

An example of my meaning has to do with my use of words – weighted according to context and theme – as Piercean signs in computer situation analysis. I was completely unaware of having developed a theoretical foundation for Kelly's Personal Construct theory until a psychologist colleague informed me of the fact.

Likewise, I have been told by an authority in the field that my use of quantitatively weighted words in this respect *is* original. Similarly, I was producing 'profiles' of both vessels and people long before the term became fashionable on television. In fact, a battery of techniques was contained in my outline design for 'User analysis ' – including the appreciation of jokes.

All such things made use of knowledge gained from earlier work into message switching in communication networks, so it is highly pertinent to this subject area. One joke, for example, could not be appreciated until the context (Editor talking to mature author)had been understood, and this context could not be understood until a script, visible backwards on a glass door, had been seen and understood.

These topics seem to be universally applicable to the process of Information Processing, and they raise questions that are similarly widely applicable. One of the questions arising is about 'practical philosophy' and how feed-back and value determination can be linked to karma and rebirth in the physical universe under psychological effects. And, to pursue this question, it helps to consider further the distinction between Platonism and mathematical Platonism.

The basic idea of a wave-front of '*Activation*' sweeping through a pre-existing framework of 'bits' of Information accentuates the differences between 'mathematical Platonism' and Platonism, per se. It also enhances both concepts while being consonant with Whitehead's Process Philosophy.

I am choosing my words carefully in using the term, 'consonant', and I do so because Plato goes *beyond* Whitehead. Readers will remember that Whitehead observed that the history of philosophy is 'nothing but a series of footnotes to Plato'. But, even Plato – after more than two thousand years - can do with updating (as Walter Mons observed about Jung's attempt to bring it about).

It follows that Plato's simile of 'the cave', in such a case, reflects characteristics of Platonism as they can be seen in the cosmological viewpoint on the physical universe, which is shown to need some amending itself. Statements, such as 'there is nothing outside the physical universe', for example, should be changed to reflect Realms, outside the physical universe, that _do_ exist but which are unobservable because of their scale.

Again, choosing my words with some care, we find that, as mathematical Platonism is advanced by modern mathematics, so Platonism is enhanced by the notions of Ideal Forms being (a) products of 'Minds' and (b) specifications of 'prescriptions and proscriptions' that are 'higher' than Mind.

My personal research and experience in such matters is reported in the Appendix and touched upon in the 'Summary/ Conclusion/ Conjectural' final part of the main body pf my argument. But, I should say here that it was initiated in methods of text-compression wherein words could be replaced in a text message by shorter numbers or other characters.

Such coding depended upon a 'dictionary' or 'lexicon', consisting of the hundred most frequently occurring words, from which a 'score' could be awarded for each context and theme considered, Based upon a grid (of Context vs. Theme), a 'response surface' could be built and used for message switching in a communications network. This most simple technique could produce text compression of up to 30%.

In real-time military operations, speed is important because data has to be kept 'fresh' – especially within a network. For example, in Aviation Technology, Symbology and Semiotics is more essential than in combat between ships because everything, in general, happens faster. This applies to a range of aircraft from huge 'jumbo jets' to fighter planes. This leads increasingly to automation, and this, in turn, leads to drones and robotics.

This tendency for ever faster decision making brings with it increased emphasis upon each symbol's clarity of meaning. In the smaller scale, pilots of aircraft (or air traffic controllers) have no time in which to puzzle out the meaning of a symbol on the screen in front of them. On a larger scale, i.e. a warship 'collective' scale, the commander in chief of a large 'combined fleet' has the same need for clarity of symbols.

To summarize and produce an 'evolutionary trail'. First, I used words as weighted signs indicating contexts and themes. I then assigned the weights according to their potency as indicators. This led to the use of words gathered together as signs pertaining especially to particular contexts and themes. Finally, three-dimensional 'response surfaces' could be produced from a basic two-dimensional grid.

It is worthy of note that an extremely simple computer program produced significant results when used to analyse human situation appraisal. Computer results could not be distinguished from those of humans. *But*, the weighting of the words was by me. However, it is not unreasonable to surmise (a) that this kind of processing could be truly evolutionary, by heuristic learning, and (b) that computers could do it.

With virtually all such advancement coming as it does from Science and Technology, and from the analogies and models made available from modern computer systems, we are obliged to consider very closely ideas pertaining to the holographic 'conjecture' or 'principle', especially as it leads us (a) into the graphical portrayals of mathematical physics, and (b) into the nature of the 'quantum vacuum'.

There is, however, a conjectural advancement that may well prove to be of greater significance and potential, and which seems custom-built for the Jung-Plato paradigm (subject to further investigation). I refer to Ervin Laszlo's 'unified field theory' which introduces a layer of organization and power into the quantum vacuum.

This notion converts immediately into the concept of a wave-front of activation sweeping through a pre-existing world of mathematics and (at the same time) removing the difficulties cited by Karl Pribram in his Foreword to *The Creative Cosmos*, which presents 'a unified science of matter, life and mind'.

Laszlo produces ideas, such as quanta being 'solitons' in an information-rich sub-quantum field, in a study which he sees as *the* [his italics] fundamental question of scientific inquiry into the nature of Reality. By definition, therefore, it overlaps with Donald MacKay's Comprehensive Reality. His 'simplest possible', when worked inot the 'Jung-Plato paradigm', produces the'simplest possible' cybernetics.

One final quotation and then I must leave this deeply interesting subject. In reference to page 178 of his book, Ervin Laszlo says:-

'Action potentials within the neural nets may be significantly affected by fluctuations in the quantum vacuum...There is now some evidence regarding the likely physiology of vacuum-triggered – that is, essentially extrasensory – signal-processing in the brain'.

And so, our thoughts fly immediately to *psychological* signal-processing, and to the *Zoharian Interface*, and to many other topics relevant to my theme. In this respect, I have to introduce the concept of 'Dualism by Properties'. This is vastly different from the concept of 'Dualism by Substance', although even this is still subject to definition. For example, the Zoharian interface is between sets of Bosons and sets of Fermions: it reduces to differences between signs, i.e. properties, but what is a *set* of subatomic particles generically? [at the same level, of course]

Although details of my experimental work have been given, I must disclose some more of its gist, here, because it is so highly pertinent. As I nudged closer to retirement, I saw that my early work on communications networks, coupled with my knowledge of Jung's 'four functions' and of measures of subjective probability, could be developed into a computer program capable of autonomic situation appraisal.

Having transmitted this 'upwards', I was given a special dispensation from the highest authorities at ASWE to continue with my work independently from the requirements of the Division. This work culminated in a carefully planned experiment –

83

over ten trials – wherein the computer evaluation of the trials could not be distinguished from the six experimental subjects.

The program was so simple, and the information given to the machine initially was so sparse, that I have no hesitation whatever in asserting that a non-human information processing system could learn by heuristic methods, *ab initio.* I will extend this to the assertion that non-living systems, i.e. robots, could do likewise.

It is noteworthy that all the psychologists among my colleagues never doubted a successful outcome to the experiment, in complete contrast to the non-psychologists who never doubted it would fail. There were also significant differences between the performances of male and female subjects, but I had no time in which to follow this up or to produce a paper from my report.

[However, it may have some significance that nearly thirty years after that report on 'Sex differences in Situation Appraisal' (13/11/14) it has just been reported (on the BBC Radio) that significant Sex differences are to be found (in outlook forecasting) on a much larger review of past statistics.]

Indeed, I can write only of techniques and methods that I have used in this field – as I have already mentioned – and these pertain either to Heuristic Learning from Signs or to an Intelligent Support System's analysis of its User. I do not claim to be the first to use the devices, but I have been told, by others better qualified in the subjects than me, that I *was* the first – and that suffices.

An example of this, however, sets the scene. It is to do with my 'weighting' of words in special 'dictionaries' according to their significance in regard of particular contexts as according to individual themes in computer analysis of situations. I was completely unaware of Kelly's Personal Construct Theory, until a psychologist colleague informed me that I had provided theoretical foundations for it. I then discovered that I had been using words as (Piercean) signs (see Elizabeth Bates).

(viii)   Input and Output

The two 'categorical varieties' of Intelligent Support System (ISS) , i.e. 'warship' and 'human', have a number of common features- as might be expected from that classification. The most basic is probably the distinction between 'raw' and 'treated' data. With raw data incoming information goes directly into its own special 'memory' wherefrom it is recovered by the various equipment needing it.

Another distinction is between input that has no urgency and input that has great urgency. In the latter case, 'ordinary' layered processing of input is waived and the pressing of an appropriate 'special purpose button' takes the processing without delay to the immediate requirement.

The checks and balances of ordinary input (in my experience) are applied in three successive layers of increasing sophistication. And, this applies to bot 'varieties of system (see Popper and Eccles). The processing takes place between communicating vessels.

Special purpose buttons are for conflict situations. MacKay (p. 58) believes they come in via 'synaptic boutons'.

So far as I was able to discern from historic design papers, the replication of a two-track input arrangement was not a deliberate copying of the brain's input processes. It may well be a general distinction applicable to all real-time action systems. It is the distinction between 'ordinary' input processing in layers of processing (see Eccles) and the operational and emergency input of Command instructions.

This latter type of input is arranged to save time, and it is achieved by having a set of 'special purpose' buttons which avoid the layers of ordinary processing and key-in, immediately, whole sets of associated sub-processes. These special groups are not dissimilar from Jung's notion of emotionally-toned 'complexes' – except, of course, that they are neurophysiological and not psychical, i.e. non-material.

There is also, in warships, a precious facility for retaining, in special, dedicated memories, certain essential data for reconfiguring the system after breakdown or serious damage. Closely similar are memories for the retention of situational data for the purposes of training, practice, rehearsal, and recreation; and, of course, the human imagination is unparalleled in this.

As automation takes hold, so will there be decreasing use of voice command input or enquiry; however there is likely to be increased use of keywords or key symbols. This, too, is common to both men and machines – especially (perhaps) in Security, Recall, and Communication.

There is one specific phenomenon which is almost – but not quite – specific to humans. I refer to the kind of 'pressure' experienced to 'get things done' – reported by John Steinbeck over the preparation of his vrsion of Arthurian legend. William James refers to a *'fiat'* from some higher system, and Rollo May is fairly closely behind. Jung deserves credit for discerning, in the first case, a 'sudden decisive impulse', and in the second case, 'hints from the unconscious'.

Pressures such as these have been called 'information pressure' which obtains in 'information mechanics'. In computer systems, they may take the form of so-called 'service streams' which offer specific details toa User. They are both powerful and demanding – special protocols and instructions _have_ to be observed; and, disaster can follow if one is abused or misused in some way.

Plato or Aristotle would probably have viewed them as superurgoi or lesser divinities or muses; and, this would have been acceptable to moderns, such as Angela Arnold, C.S. Lewis, and Danah Zohar (I feel). Jung, Steinbeck, and countless others, would have recognized 'daimons' at work.

Finally, there are many *internal* subconscious or *'periconscious'* (i.e. real-time but not conscious) processes seeking attention and 'need-satisfaction'. Some of these operate in parallel with autonomous functions, which can be 'hard-wired', and, for maintainers, repairers, Users, et al., they need to be identified and _documented_. [It is a somewhat daunting thought that if some kind of system of rebirth is operational for humans such things must exist in regard of living processes.]

In this respect, we are perhaps given hope by the fact that in the warship *everything* from operating system and search engine to the smallest component – is built-up from the simplest of components, such as clocks, timers, 'flags', lists, rotas, interrupts, etc., etc. Ernest Kent makes this point; and Donald MacKays puts it into practice.

(ix) Hierarchies of Networks and Nodes

At this point, I introduce an author who has gradually fought his way to recognition – if not complete acceptance.   Many moons ago, he burst on the scientific scene and caused the Editor of Nature, no less, to declare that his book should be burned [I never dreamed I'd ever see that day].   Since then, his ideas have become cited by the most eminent scientists and clerics (but not necessarily endorsed).

I refer, of course, to Dr. Rupert Sheldrake, whose notion of morphogenetic fields (and its corollaries) is proving apposite to the ideas of mathematical Platonism, in general, and to the Axis of Scale, in particular.   Sheldrake's book, *The Science* Delusion, contains one of the few diagrammatic representation of hierarchical 'nesting' along the axis that I have seen.   It is still, however, open to misinterpretation (see *The Science Delusion*, page 50).

Sheldrake's central theme is that there are so-called 'morphogenetic fields', whose name identifies their function.   He debunks the Richard Dawkins concept of Evolution (correctly, in my opinion) and produces a figure illustrating the hierarchical nesting of entities, giving examples across differing fields of interest and research.

The diagram is nominated as representing nested hierarchies of wholes, but the concept of a 'whole' would probably be considered by others as 'parts'.   So, care must be taken over terminology.   My examples of the hierarchical grouping of warships, and of the parallel growth of extended knowledge and communication systems, might be acceptable to Rupert Sheldrake; but, it would not be welcomed from all quarters.   For example, the current 'easing out' of Jung's 'Racial Unconscious' seems, to me, caused entirely by political correctness.

A number of features of Sheldrake's theories, however, *do* seem to overlap somewhat with the characteristics of the Jung-Plato paradigm.   In addition to those already listed, there are warm references to Whitehead, to minds 'extended' in Time, and to another way of thinking about 'wholes', i.e. systems theory.

He points out that systems theory speaks of 'a configuration of parts joined together by a web of relationships', but such wholes are often called 'complex systems', which are the subject of a number of mathematical models called variously 'complex systems theory', 'complexity theory', or 'complexity science' (p. 51).

Sheldrake backs up his notions with examples, and I like particularly his description of a crystal lattice as 'a nested hierarchy of levels of organization interacting through a nested hierarch of vibrating fields'.   I rather like, also, his discussion of Telepathy and Clairvoyance presented in another book, *The Sense of Being Stared At*.

Be that as it may, in my opinion, Sheldrake provides in his books a good illustration of (a) the need for an epitheoretic organization of information into Orders and Degrees according to their value re contexts and themes (i.e. subjective probability and, perhaps, other things such as Radical Pragmatism) and (b) a requirement for the science that he so abjures to concentrate more (rather than less) upon the case for mechanism and determinism (while still allowing for Freedom of Will).

In other words, Sheldrake's ideas are more suited to the discovery or unveiling of existing 'truths' than to the emergence of 'new' truths.   His argument for Emergence is based upon a philosophy of organism that is rooted in whitehead's process philosophy and the conjecture that the cosmos is a developing organism (2013, pp. 48-55).

Process philosophy, however worthy (and I use it as a sounding board), is just a set of conjectures.   It seems to me dubious that it should be in-built as part of an argument; and one certainly cannot take it for granted that the cosmos is a developing organism.

Science needs original thinkers, such s Rupert Sheldrake, but 'methinks he does protest too strongly, and wildly, and shallowly' (pace Shakespeare – I thought it the most appropriate comment).   At a time when Science is rendering it increasingly difficult to distinguish between living and non-living organisms – and producing more and more 'hybrid' systems – his arguments, on those counts, seem (to me) strangely out of date.   I will add to this comment, later.

(x) Processes and Stories

This vein of thought in the previous subsection leads one to the simplest and most just system of thought that can be imagined – short of hard-line or extreme determinism. I refer to the melding or merger of mathematical Platonism with Donald MacKay's Comprehensive Reality re the proposed Jung-Plato paradigm.

MacKay's scheme of Mechanistic Embodiment accords with this paradigm completely except for his notion that an organism is the embodied mathematical formula, e.g. a set of differential equations (see von Bertalanffy) held only in the mind of God.

However, following the lead of my (mathematical) betters, I have that formula (i.e. Ideal Form) also represented in a region of 'etheriality' that exists 'just within' the physical universe' [this is a notion no worse, in my opinion, than 'the empty set'.   It fits with many other notions.]

The 'embodiment' in question takes the form of a 'wave-front' (in the customary sense) of *activation* sweeping through the 'world' of mathematics.   The wave-front, however, does not collapse – it is as if a 'hand' brushes a set of beads in an immense abacus.   The simile is not too dissimilar from Plato's 'shadows on a cave wall' simile.

The 'organism' or 'Action System', resulting from the embodiment, is equally simple.   It is bifid – there are just two functionaries and two corresponding processes. One such process is the n-dimensional body driven by an _Agent_ responsible for *everything* concerning the past present and future; and a _Determinator_, which selects the best *action alternative* for its purpose or Mission.

There are numerous pertinent facors supporting this basic simplicity.   In no particular order of precedence, they are:-

(a) As I write, certain physicists are conjecturing a mathematical function that 'drives' the 'cosmos' in the ways I describe, including the complex plane extension. (See Matthew Chalmers).

(b) The 'Determinator' function is reducible to a number of specialisms within the Agent, _but,_ as Bertrand Russell is reported to have said, 'the existence of a loosely conjoined aggregate of powers does not necessarily mean that there is no simple soul or *atman'* (Huxley, p. 136).

(c) Everything is consistent with the concept of humans being 'characters in stories' and, in the picture I have just sketched out, a person or, more likely, a relationship can be taken back exactly, as in karma, to the point at which he/she/they made the serious error of judgment.

(d) In this scenario, Plato would have individuals or 'poles' of a relationship intuiting the Good, Truth, etc., and MacKay would simply have them being 'free' to differ from their 'story' – the quality or value of their choice would be, of course, up to them.

(e) The _Mission_, for Plato, would be re-union outside the physical universe; and MacKay allows for union, merger, indwelling, of systems.

(f) Writing on the philosophy of language, philosopher, Mark Platts, discusses 'ethical intuitionism' in which the object of intuition is 'The Good'. He admits the existence of *many* (his emphasis) distinct ethical qualities – honesty, sincerity, loyalty, etc. – and sees no reason to assume *a priori* that they cannot conflict (pp. 244-7).

(g) Clearly, subjective probability, categorization, hierarchy, and so on have relevance in this, and many other subjects, and it is open to conjecture that some 'epitheoreticl network' could or should obtain.

Finally, there is one special set of ideas that, I feel, should be investigated – that is the notion of Interaction between fields.   The 'partly-baked' idea of interaction between fields of force and fields of information was first introduced in 1964 by Cyril Burt (see *The Scientist Speculates)*, Ed. I.J. Good).

This coincided with the arrival of computers and their Users, and it happened to coincide, loosely, with Sherrington's analogy of genuine interaction between the sun and his elbow.   This, I mention to illustrate a radical difference between the concepts of interaction.   A difference, I might add, that still leads to misconceptions and errors.

Even when a 'computer' has been given a sophisticated and powerful operating system, there is no interaction between the computer and its User in the sense that Sherrington meant. The 'computer' with that kind of operating system is an 'Intelligent Support System' that is part of the Action System (i.e. 'organism'), but it only *communicates* with its User.

Sherrington's interaction had the sun acting physically upon his elbow and his elbow acting physically upon the sun – although, of course, indetectably. Popper and Eccles grasped this, in part. They had the user system (wrongly identified as the programmer) 'writing to' and 'reading from' the computer (system) but they failed to demonstrate how the system acts back physically onto the User or the programmer. And, of course, they could not do so.

Ernest Kent and Donald MacKay, in their various ways, showed that there is no need for such a genuine interaction. In fact, since Sherrington, technology has advanced so much that we can conceive quite easily of 'hybrid' action systems, per se, reading and writing from 'scripts' (for want of a better word) and experiencing very strong *feelings* of being characters in stories.

MacKay believed an individual human organism (an embodied Action system or formula) to be a character in a story having only limited freedom of action, i.e. to act differently from the action decreed in the 'script' or written story. [For Donald MacKay, this was the Bible - see his *Freedom of Action in a Mechanistic Universe*.]

However, this is immaterial [no pun intended] – we are concerned with the actions and behaviour, generally, of a material system acting out a 'story' that is prescribed (and proscribed in an Ideal Form) in a universe consisting (so it is thought) only of relationships and fields. And, today, there are numerous examples of how two different *kinds* of fields can affect and influence each other.

Leaving many side-issues aside, this simple, bald statement reaches out into very many pertinent) regions of thought. For example, it intrudes into the 'solenoid model' (fact) and the Yin and Yang principles (theory), and into the 'Zoharian Interface' between sets of Bosons and sets of Fermions fact/theory).

Critically, such arguments (as I understand them) set Platt's notion of 'intuitional morality', supported by Jungian theory and Platonic theory, against Sheldrake's interpretation of process philosophy (garnered from one book by Whitehead and two books *on* Whitehead) which seems to accept metaphysical assertion as fact. However, this kind of discussion takes us outside the physical universe – where there is nothing, according to Lee Smolin.

No one (I hope) would call me an 'Establishment man', but it seems to me that Rupert Sheldrake's diatribe against Science, in *The Science Delusion,* is shallow and facile. He presents, so to speak, a series of dots which are in need of being joined up. Mathematical Platonism, accompanied by Comprehensive Realism and the Sino-Asiatic model and a reconstructed Jungian Theory, does the 'joining up' impeccably.

I can illustrate my meaning by reference to Sheldrake's use of Whitehead's notion of basic 'events' being 'occasions of experience'. This concept is quite consonant with many other schemes of thought which could be regarded as 'dots' to be joined up.

For example, the 'dots' could be mathematical Platonism, Comprehensive Reality, the Sino-Asiatic model, particle physics, and the suggested 'Jung-Plato paradigm, which sees 'occasions of experience' as a wave-front of activation sweeping through the world of mathematics. Or, a collection of 'stories' written by either one single Author or a number of Contributors (both under Editorial constraints).

Covering all these things, and more, we have very wise words from physicist, Gary Zukav. His book, *The Dancing Wu Li Masters*, has been called 'an excellent guide into the magic of modern physics'. The pertinence can be assessed by the words of David Finklestein (pp. 330-2), who says:-

'I think it would be misleading to call particles the entities involved in the most primitive events of the theory [quantum topology] because they don't move in space and time, they don't carry mass, they don't have charge, they don't have energy in the usual sense of the word'.

From another perspective, Zukav explains (p. 300) that 'Buddhism is both a philosophy and a practice. Buddhist philosophy is rich and profound. Buddhist practice is called *Tantra*. *Tantra* is the Sanscript word meaning "to weave". There is little that can be said about *Tantra*. It must be done'. And, we can reflect about the closeness of the concept of *Tantra* to the assertion by Rollo May that Love contains a Command imperative to Act.

Gary Zukav is referring to a 'level' which is similar to the 'hidden geometry' containing the power and elegance of 'certain abstract symmetries' associated with the geometry of extra dimensions of space – when regarded from a viewpoint somewhat 'higher' than that of Zukav. That is to say, from a viewpoint which weaves together space, time, and matter into a 'unified field' (see Davies, 1987, pp. 160-1).

It is difficult to see why Rupert Sheldrake is so vehement about modern science from comparisons like these. Science seems to be doing a pretty good job in producing the same kind of 'Truth' from differing perspectives. I think that his vehemence may be caused by his confusing Platonism with *mathematical Platonism* and by his *selective* reading of Lee Smolin.

Regarding the former, anyone wishing to understand *Platonism* could do worse than consult *Plato*, by R.M. Hare, and *mathematical Platonism* by consulting *The Road to Reality*, by Roger Penrose. For *mathematical Intuition and mysticism*, Rudy Rucker's *Infinity and the Mind* is admirable. It is noteworthy that one can hardly view *any* proposition of Plato's without taking one of a number of 'perspectives'.

In fact, there is a difference between making a 'fair' case and making a case that is unbalanced and misrepresents a situation. In my opinion, Sheldrake's argument against Science is 'biased' – in the same sense that Jung's ideology was biased. In other words, it is biased in the statistical sense of the term. For example, his attack on Science contains no mention of anything mentioned in my last paragraph (excluding particularly *Mysticism*.

In *THREE ROADS TO QUANTUM GRAVITY*, Lee Smolin describes how the flow of information around the circuits of a computer constitutes a story in which events are computations and causal processes are just the flow of bits of information from one computation to the next.

He portrays, in short, a *relational universe of events* – begging the question 'Are not occasions of experience events? Moreover, Smolin devotes a whole chapter 'How to *weave* a string (my emphasis).

Furthermore, he points out that, under certain principles, 'the world must be a network of holograms, each of which contains coded within it information about the relationships between the others. In short, the *holographic principle* is the " ultimate realization of the notion that the world is a network of relationships"…revealed to involve nothing but information' (p. 178).

This takes us to yet another matter of possible bias. In this case, the bias is in terms of mathematical preferences and their relation to Mysticism. It relates to the 'Holographic principle', as it is called by Lee Smolin, and the 'Holographic Conjecture', as it is called more cautiously by Roger Penrose.

In this case, however, the matter is of more consequence, because – sold as a 'principle – it opens the 'flood gates', as it were, to all kinds of 'fringe' (to put it mildly) ideas and 'the usual suspects' come pouring in. The difficulty, brought in thus, is that – almost by definition - there should be more than a grain of truth behind some of the ideas.

Dr. Smolin's use of the word 'information', coupled with his lack of references to process philosophy (when discussing events and processes), triggers a response in me of doubt. He defines the term as 'a measure of information about a signal – this measure being equal to the number of Yes/No questions whose answers could be coded in the signals'.

This, alone, gives me unease, because the questions, if phrased in natural language, cannot be posed without given supplementary information about contexts, themes, and kinds (of information). In short, natural language is not sufficient for the job. The use of any other language reduces the argument.

There are, also, other reasons for doubt. For example, systems theorists would argue strongly against the ideas of the physical universe being a closed system with *nothing* outside it. It is a tenet of systems theory that all systems have environments.

We can, and we should, thank William Johnston for helping us, amid this welter of ideas, to *discern* at least the semblance of truth and logic as it pertains to the Jung-Plato paradigm. Geared to the phenomena of the material Realm, Dr. Johnston explains to us how experience and *experience of knowledge* can be achieved in mystical union, merger, and, especially, *indwelling*.

He points out that Buddhism and Christianity are step by step consonant with each other up to the point of mystical union with Jesus Christ. That is to say, I suggest, within the physical universe; and, that allows me to introduce what I call (loosely) the phenomena of 'lay mysticism'.

Ursula King, in *Towards a New Mysticism*, describes how Teilhard de Chardin makes much the same distinction in (a) his differentiation between 'roads' of the East and of the West and (b) the *experience of knowledge*. The latter, we conjecture, is more easily understood when Jung's functions of Intuition and Feeling are brought together as I have indicated.

Dr. King, in fact, links a 'New Mysticism of Action' to Jung and to Whitehead, and she envisages a 'battle of the spirit' necessary today in the conflict between a 'religious and a humanistic-atheistic worldview' (p. 225), Beyond such needs, however, Ursula King sees a 'pressing task for world religions to engage in dialogue with contemporary culture'. [In other words, for them to take on 'the social Leviathan']

In this, I am touching upon those 'extra-sensory' ways of information transfer of the kind, for example, identified by J.B. Priestley and described within a mass of detritus by Michael Talbot in *The Holographic Universe*. [An example of what I mean is given in a half-dozen or so pages on 'Instantaneous knowledge', in which emotion and knowledge are shown as being pre-eminent in the 'afterlife dimension' (?!).]

Although I have used chess notation to indicate the term to be questionable, it *does* have a ring of truth to it. It ties in with everyday experience, in the sense (the Priestley sense) that occasions of knowledge so-gained are more commonplace than we realize. For example, and speaking as a statistician, both my daughter and I have experience of the instantaneous and/or precognitive acquisition of knowledge that is far, far beyond the limits of coincidence.

Modern real-time computer systems have such powers that the concepts of the intercommunication of experiential knowledge has no mystery, and is 'to be expected' from many kinds of computer analogies. I have in mind, as I write, the kind of discussion offered by Rudy Rucker, in 'Infinity *and the Mind'* wherein he muses upon robots and their souls and dimensions.

More pragmatically, but no less philosophical, the technicalities of 'bounds' and 'limits' along the Axis of Scale (Rucker's 'dimension' of scale) are thrown into prominence through the holographic implications given by Smolin (pp. 169-178). This involves an interpretation of Platonism that appears to be confounded with mathematical Platonism, from which I bow out.

(xi)   Individuation, Command, Leadership, Specialization

Covered in Part Three

(xii)   Natural Mind

Part Three

(xiii)   Embodiment and Recorded Material

Part Three

(xiv)   Categorization of Contexts and Themes

Part Three

(xv)   Systems Malfunctions and Disturbances

In this respect, I am acutely conscious of the plethora of books on mental illness or unbalance and similarities to computer performance.   For example, Ludwig von Bertalanffy discusses this topic over some seventeen pages (pp217-234) in his *General System Theory*.

In his *Robots, Men and Minds,* he devotes three pages to the close resmblances of 'normal' brain functioning to similar processes in a computer (pp. 99-101).   He points out that there is no 'sharp' borderline between bodily function and the conscious mind and unconscious mind.

As he says, physiological function in behaviour and neurophysiology increasingly begin to resemble psychological function (conscious and unconscious) in their *structural* aspects.   He, then, spends several pages on on the ways in which simple components resemble each other and how assemblies of such components are similar, too.   His conclusion is that ultimately body and mind may prove to be just one system.

In that respect, therefore, I am merely expanding upon that theme – but I am not, im any way, suggesting an identity between mind and <u>soul</u>.   In terms of function, 'mind' is the functioning and identities produced by the material brain/Mind(Ego), and 'Soul' is (probably) a physical system that is NOT material.

Therefore, with no psychiatric knowledge implied, I offer the following 'possibles' for consideration.

(a)   Key Words

These are used in a number of ways, and they can be of considerable importance – particularly in matters of System Integrity or Security (e.g. of System, Vessel, or Mission). In humans, key words might relate to merely past enjoyable experiences, but equally they might pertain to Guilt, Phobias, Ambitions, Fears, Conscience, as well as to 'Suppression', 'Repression', 'Hypnosis', and 'Parapraxex'.

Some particular examples from warship experience are (possibly) 'Hysterical Paralysis', 'Catatonia', 'Nervous Breakdown', Mannerisms and idiosyncrasies, 'Amnesia', 'Fixation', and 'Complexes'.

(b) Freezing ('Hysterical Paralysis', Seizures, 'Catatonia', Hypnosis)

This condition seems applicable, in general, to the higher animals. It occurs when no input can be made to the Intelligent Support System through the keyboards of VDUs (or touch pads, light pens, or whatever), and it results in partial or complete breakdown of the whole action system – no command or control signal can be entered. The condition can be induced in rats by blasts of high pressure air being released and it is unmistakable (but the practice is brutal).

Modern systems *should* be designed to avoid this fault, which seems usually to be caused by 'overload' conditions unforeseen by the designers, [Techniques with laboratory rats were intiated in the 1950s (about the time of Lashley). Although remarkably successful they, too, were discontinued as being too brutal] With computer systems, the only way to restore system dynamics may sometimes be to shut down the whole system and then to 'boot it up again'.

(c) Ghosts (Hallucinations, Hypnotic States)

'Ghosts' arise in the warship on the screens of VDUs much as they can on domestic television. Weather conditions *can* produce them or sunspot activity, or human carelessness in more local conditions. For example, a carelessly placed magnetic in the computer room will cause them – often in the form of marvellously intricate patterns in the style of William Morris. In humans, medical drugs, such as certain antibiotics will produce similar but more varied effects. However, there is no continuity or coherence such as in ESP.

As I have already mentioned, a particularly notable feature is that the 'operations room' of an operational warship, with its dim lighting, glittering screens of differing performances and symbologies, is quite strongly reminiscent of various psychological descriptions of mental activity and hypnagogic imagery.

A human being has no display screen in his/her mind, as is pointed out by Donald MacKay, but there do exist a score or more 'visual areas' in the brain which are integrated into a number odf matrices which serve as 'pictures' for the appropriate processes (MacKay, 1991, p. 91).

Popper and Eccles asserted that 'the ghost in the machine' *is* an appropriate term for a 'User system', despite their critics, but their claims appear to be justified only by a dualism by properties. Their description of the brain as a form of computer support system is, however, excellent; and its activities include processes for 'looking ahead' and 'preparing' sub-systems for immanent action. The 'Ops. Room' analogy, to which I refer, corresponds also to the number of 'specialist' subsystems in the brain.

(d) The Deadly Embrace (Breakdown, Apathy, Boredom)

This is well known in computer circles. Doubtless, because of its striking and graphic title. But it *does* seem likely to have an underlying mechanism which might be shared with human frailties. It is cased often by a design fault which has been described famously as 'Process P waiting for Procee Q waiting for Process P' (Djikstra). The symptoms are that the system either becomes unbalanced or becomes inert – depending upon the nature of the system and/or the capability of the designer. In yesterday's culture it provided a 'Catch 22 situation', but it still occurs today.

(f) Thrashing (Breakdown, Frenzy)

The symptoms occur at moments when processes are competing for time or space in the main processor. M.V. Wilkes went into this problem long ago and formally. It lies in the province of Control Engineering. Wilkes discovered that Thrashing may occur in the same way as the Deadly Embrace, i.e. in the seekig of optimal performance in the usage of core-memory or in time-sharing. Absence of thrashing in a proposed system can be proved theoretically. The phenomenon, therefore, can be regarded as an indication of either poor design or system malfunction.

(g) Over-Alertness (Anxiety, Mannerisms, 'Fixations', Idiosyncrasy)

This is often seen in the performance of equipment that is obsolescent or superseded in part, and it is caused by pieces not having been properly removed or blanked-off. The outcome is an intermittent and unwarranted influence that impairs effectiveness. Examples are to be found in the erratc running of things like weapon platforms or missile launchers or sensors.

The normally smooth running is interrupted by a brief hesitation or acceleration. Other examples are, when in threat evaluation, certain targets may be given unwarranted amounts of attention or priority status. The phenomenon could, and should, be taken as a warning against 'patching' or 'quick fixes' of programs rather than re-writing them. To a lay observer, the occurrences may seem like a nervous tic.

(h) (System Imbalances (esp. Extraversion; Introversion)

I have already referred to states such as these in which pre-set parameters are exceeded. In general, these 'out of limits' polarities are caused by unduly heavy or unduly light weightings given to assessments of priority or of significance in other ways, such as allowances of space or of time. Extraversion and Introversion pertain to matters of 'balancing' the processes that are either 'internal' or 'external' regarding an entity and its environment.

This is comparatively easy when the entity is an organism, but more complicated when the entity is an operating system. In this case, the entity (i.e. the operating system) might be regarded as the *'Agent'* and its environment considered to be 'the rest of the organism' (i.e. the *'Determinator'*). This is the terminology used by Donald MacKay in his scheme of mechanistic embodiment.

In a warship, the limits will have been set either by the designer of the system or by the Commander of the warship for some special operational reason. Today, it is likely that more modern designers are building in processes by which its specialized subsystems can generate its own limits by heuristic learning in regard of contexts, themes, and results.

Such a capacity, in humans, would be part of the brain's development from the brain stem , early limbic system, etc., along the evolutionary trail as the 'lower' systems of the brain develop the operating system apace with the higher functions of Perception and Judgment. The issue of limits might just relate to the 'principles of limitations' conjectured by Whitehead.

(xvi) Defence Mechanisms

On this issue, I am acutely conscious of being still under the Official Secrets Act – clearly I cannot reveal any aspects of a warship's defence mechanisms. However, I am writing about the very earliest of 'Intelligent Support Systems', about 'composite' systems, about systems that exist only in outline on paper (and will never be built), so these things, added to my discretion, allow me to disclose with confidence that a warship's defences are every bit as deep, wide-spread, and difficult to penetrate, as are a human being's.

In Jungian terms, the Shadow, the Persona, and other material that is 'secret', all overlap. To illustrate this, I will quote something I wrote decades ago and is as relevant today as it was then. Throughout, it will be seen that there is much scope (and necessity) for _Keywords_, for _Symbolism_, and for _Imagery_ , and it is all applicable to the natural mind, i.e. to the Brain and its Mind(Ego):-

'These 'shadowy' areas include attention to Security of Knowledge, Security of Vessel, Security of Mission, Security of Itinerary, Avoidance of Danger (to Mission and to Vessel), Masking Vessel's Identity, Protection of Facilities for Recovery from Damage or Breakdown, Monitoring and Maintaining System Performance, Promulgating Real and False Identities/Intentions, Safeguarding Self and Others, etc., etc.'

(xvii) Trickery and Guile

Jung thought this matter sufficiently important to call it an 'archetype', i.e. the _Trickster_. He was wrong to do so, because the Trickster is just one pole of many relationships with the category of _Victim_. [Zoharian philosophy would have a whole sub-category having a combined effect upon one individual]. Moreover, the phenomena of trickery and guile is far, far lower down the evolutionary trail than the 'social Leviathan'. Almost back to the protozoan, one might think.

Notions of 'profiles' and 'signatures' are commonplace today, as are Victims and 'Suckers (i.e. the most gullible). The art of 'feigning' and 'dissembling' , to which politicians are particularly given, is an extremely primitive one [how apt] and a warship's manipulation of its electromagnetic radiation to mislead a foe is a very similar process.

The process has reached a high level of Security classification _and of Secrecy_ (not, perhaps, the highest, but not far off), and so I will say no more on that subject. However, a moment's thought indicates that human trickery and guile certainly go back to the times of Homer. In fact, the 'Trojan Horse' is an appropriate name in use some three thousand years on.

(xviii) The Taxonomic Position

It is no 'big deal' to point out the closeness between the human and the warship in these matters. However, there is obviously confusion about the so-called 'mind-body problem'; and it is high time that this preoccupation and loose talk about it were removed.

Within a so-called scientific approach to this problem, we have a ridiculous situation wherein one group of eminent scientists assert that the brain's whole neural network answers to no 'Command element' (i.e. that which gives the *fiat*), and the other group flatly contradicts that assertion. Both sets appear to be wrong and both sets are not only *indisputably* making a metaphysical assertion, but also hypostatizing it (see Jung's *Memories, Dreams, Reflections*).

In such a situation, I resort to systems theory backed up by subjective probability and measure my opinions against Whitehead's Process Philosophy (strictly as a 'sounding board', because it is completely conjectural).

However, this can be improved. I say this because an error that transcends and includes the misconceptions of the rival factions is that of *'wrong categorization'*. Ludwig von Bertalanffy addresses this (1967 and 1973), and I have shown, in *Automation and Sex Differences in Situation Appraisal,* how this can happen in human cases.

Amid a proliferation of terms lacking definition we have 'soul', 'spirit', 'psyche', and 'mind' – or so it seems. They all have meaning within the parameters of some particular faction or other. W.E.R. Mons writes well on this subject, and he pleads for patience with Jung because of the difficulties of translation.

However, they *do* slot into place when we trace their position by treating *Scale* as a dimension (as is suggested by Rudy Rucker) and following the evolutionary path of organismic development along the axis of scale. In this respect, the writer L.L. Whyte predicted (more than hald a century ago) that one day *body* and *mind* would be regarded as 'one conceptual system'.

Ludwig von Bertalanffy makes that point when averring that mental disease is essentially a disturbance of systems functions in the psychophysical organism' (p. 230). But, what exactly does 'psychophysical' mean?. Freud and Jung would have given different answers to that question.

It helps the understanding of all these terms if we consider a taxonomy of system types. Study of this reveals just how close man is to machine in this respect:-

Order	General Systems
Family	Information Processing
Genus	Real-Time I-P
Species	Adaptive, User Supportive R-T, I-P
Sub-Speies	User-Analytical, Self-Adaptive, R-T, I-P
Variety	Human, Computer, Hybrid, U-A, S-A, R-T, I-P

(xix) Preparations for Action

(a) Preparing Action Alternatives

Ernest Kent asserts that the ability to make perceptual feed-forward projections in the context of goal-directed decision-making is the defining characteristic of a 'High Command' within the brain (p. 194). His knowledge of computer hardware and software may be part of his 'considerable experience', but real-time Intelligent Support Systems are clearly outside his mind-ser, i.e. knowledge base.

I say this because of his terminology. The term 'High Command' reflects a function several levels of authority above that of the part of an organism which 'gives the nod', so to speak, to the ISS to proceed with its suggested action. It is part of the Support System's design to suggest a preferred option to the superordinate system; and in Donald MacKay's organismic scheme of Comprehensive Realism the two subsystems of the organism, respectively, are dubbed 'the Agent' and 'the Determinator'.

We have to bear in mind, however, that the 'nod' to which I refer is a *fiat* given by a subsystem of a material organism that lies in other dimensions of the physical world. William James, the Victorian, used the term for such a realm as being *'superconscious'* and this term has been used by others more recently (see J.B. Priestley)

This having been said, Kent's *The Brains of Men and Machines* makes an excellent companion to Donald MacKay's *Behind the EYE* in regard of the 'brain/mind(Ego)' being a support system. In my opinion, Ernest Kent misunderstands the 'supervisor' function in this respect.

(b) Preparing for Action (Pre-firing of Circuits)

There are many analogies between man and machine in regard of preparing for action in the material world – deliberate, unconscious, and autonomous. Anyone knowledgeable about the seamier side of life could testify that an awareness of preliminary signs of 'trouble' may lead to the avoidance of serious personal harm.

However, in my chosen context the isomorphism is clear and simple, and, although mechanistic, it is initiated by knowledge. I refer to a mechanism common to both warship and human being. That is to say, armed with that knowledge, in both kinds of organism, there is a preliminary firing of neural circuits that will be used in a forthcoming action. The purpose is twofold: first, the pre-firing alerts the circuits and, so to speak, warms them up, and second it checks their availability and functionality.

(xx) Information Gathering and Retrieval Errors

It is in this area that man and machine seem to come closest together in various forms of parapraxis. Erroneous information is usually caused by either faulty retrieval from relational associative memory, or by faults in the 'next item' addresses contained within a single item of data.

Relational and/or associative memory is storage in which there is a redundancy in the storage of data – in comparison with other methods of storage – in order to save time or for some other form of expediency . To counter-balance this excess, items of information are sometimes 'chained' together higgledy-piggledy.

[I must confess that my machine code programs were often stored in this fashion – which is alright if the program is correct or nearly developed but introduces difficulties otherwise.] Alternatively, wrong addresses may be given to the search engine seeking data retrieval, or in the delivery to the User from the search engine.

Errors of this kind are probably more common in 'liveware' or 'wetware' than in non-living 'hardware', but in all cases information can be revealed which could prove embarrassing or, even, disastrous. On the other hand, they could lead to mutual amusement or even friendship. For example, I once asked a pretty young girl assistant in a bookshop for Kimsey's 'Human Behaviour in the Sexual Female', which caused instant merriment and rapport between us.

On the other hand, slips of the tongue _do_ often have the potential for disaster, and I can recall how disaster was narrowly averted at the end of a long hard day (apparently) by the manger of a wine shop. I was behind a lady, waiting to be served, who was being exceedingly perverse and irritating even to me – she really was impossible.

The manager was containing his impatience admirably, but he was clearly anxious to wind up business for the day. His female customer had been besieging him for some time with stupid questions and vapid side-issues, and I repeat the incident verbatim – because both were considerably older than me and they are both probably dead.

She finally got round to paying for her quite small order and she asked if she could pay by cheque. The manager, keeping his cool, replied 'Certainly, Madam', and then came her final affront. Having received his assent, she wrote as he spoke, spelling out the name – letter by letter. The name, letter by leter, was given her as 'Somebody or Other, Cow'.

What a difference one letter can make! Fortunately for him, she was so self-important that she didn't notice his Freudian slip. He realized immediately what he had done, and looked appalled. He caught my eye, and I winked sympathetically to indicate that I shared his opinion.

For my penultimate task as an RN scientist I was requested to produce an outline specification for a putative real-time computer system capable of analysing its User and of adapting itself to his 'profile' if it were found to be 'off-limits'. The report is in three parts and is entered in the Bibliography. It went into the User's understanding of jokes; and it would have needed just the kind of semantic web that is being developed today. And so, this seems an excellent opportunity for proceeding to Part Three, which addresses such things.

PART THREE: GLOSSARY AND GUIDE

INTRODUCTION

This Part of the proffered Jung-Plato paradigm identifies some of the 'nodes' in the 'web or network' of concepts – philosophical and scientific – that underlies the approach of any scientist seeking to establish the underlying roots of his/her discipline. Clearly each and every scientist undertaking the exercise will develop his/her individual personal web or network either initially or by upon the one which follows.

However, the methodology is closely associated with personal construct theory (see APPENDIX) and the creation of 'nodes' and the linking of them together can be used in a number of different ways in different contexts for different purposes. Additionally, various analytical techniques can be developed for learning and synthesizing material in this way.

The networks and their nodes are entirely malleable.   Indeed, as knowledge is gained it would be expected that the categories would be changed or re-named and that fresh ones would be introduced.

My main ain in this monograph is to support the case for evolutionary psychology by showing that Personality is a product of the functioning brain.   This, I believe is done in Part Two, beyond reasonable doubt.   Part Three is aimed primarily at showing how unity of thought – between nations, disciplines, individual people – _could_ be achieved by the power of computer networks specially designed for the purpose.

Each entry illustrates the deep complexity of ideas underlying its derivation and meaning – as a concept.   However, as I have said in the text, Part Three is not only exemplary but is also ephemeral.   In computer-talk it (or something like it) is for the on-line gathering of, and improving upon, Information.   It will change as this process continues and the process is 'open ended'

With clarity of exposition at heart, I have left some of the items indicated but not developed.   As in Part Two, I hope this is sufficient, and I have tried to compensate to some extent by making the Bibliography as helpful as possible to readers.   However, I have seized the opportunity, with certain items, to expand upon material of Part Two which, if included in that Part, might have obfuscated or clouded the drift of my argument.

LIST OF NODES OR ENTRIES

Abbreviations and Acronyms, Agents, Altered States of Consciousness, Anima/Animus, Anthropic Perspective, Aristotle, Artificial Intelligence, Attention, Attractors and Strange Attractors, Awareness, Axis of Scale, Bennett's Mathematical Model, Body of Belief, Boundaries, Carrying Over, Categorisation, Causality, Central Order, Clairvoyance, Clinical Tools, Cohomology, Cold Dark Matter, Command Fiat, Comprehensive Reality, Common Sense, Computer Systems, Connectors, Consciousness, Contexts and Themes, Cosmic Parochialism, Cosmological Influences and Effects, Data and Reality, de Sitter space, Decision-making, Delgado, Demiurgoi, Diagrammatic Representation, Dimensions, Dimensional Time, Dualism, Elective Affinity, Encephalized Mind(Ego), Engine Driver, Entanglement, Epitheoretical Analysis, Etheriality, Evidence, Evil, Experience, Free Will, Freudian Theory, Gravitational Effects, Grids, Profiles, Truth, Health, Heuristic Learning, Hidden Dimensions, Hierarchy, Higgs Boson, Hinduism, Holistic Dualism, Holistic Relationism, Holographic Principle, Hypothesis of Duality, 'I', Ideal Forms, Identities and Selves, Implementation and Manifestation, Individuation, Indwelling and Merger, Inexplicable Features, Inner Self, Isomorphism, Jungian Theory, Karma and Rebirth, Life Force, Loop Quantum Gravity, Love and Sex, Mission and Command, Moral Responsibility, Manifestation and Implementation, Moving Finger, Mystical Knowledge (& ESP), Mystical Language and Communications, Myths and Irrationality, Natural Philosophy, Natural Quaternion, Nature's Aim, Networks and Nodes, Noble Eightfold Path, Ockham's Razor, Operating Systems, Order of Magnitude, Pantheism and Panentheism, Passions, Perspectivism, Pilot, Platonic World, Plausibility, Plurality of Consciousness, Pontifical Nerve-cell, Priestley, Primacy, Principle of Convergence, Process, Process Image/Ideal Form, Process Philosophy, Programs and Stories, Propensity, Psychagogues, Purpose, Quantumchromodynamics (QCD), Quantum Relational Holism, Quartic Organum, Quintic Organum, Quaternions, Rankian Theory, Relationism, Relational Holism, Reflection Principle, Riemannian Geometry, Robotics and Computation, Sapientia, Scale, Self, Self-Discovery, Sentics, Service Stream, Set Theory, Sex and Love, social Leviathan, Soul, Spin, Spin Networks, Spirit, Strong Dualistic Hypothesis, Subjective Probability, Superconscious, Subordinacy and Superordination, Superintelligence, Superstrings, Supersymmetry, Supervisor, Systems Theory, Taxonomy, Teilhard, The Way, Theism, Torus, Triune Brain & Triagic mind(Ego), Truth, Twistor Theory, Veils and Voids, Visions and Personifications, Warship Analogy, Weight of Evidence, World Line, Yin-Yan Co-operation, Zoharian Interface.

INDIVIDUAL ENTRIES

ABBREVIATIONS AND ACRONYMS

AGENT

The term 'Agent' is commonplace and applied to quite widely differing entities – so definition is required. In Donald MacKay's scheme of Comprehensive Reality the Agent is that part of an embodied mathematical formula which maintains an operational organismal body and prepares sets of future action alternatives for the organism.

A recommended action is offered to the 'Determinator', and this 'Command element' (i.e. Sherrington's 'ultimate pontifical nerve cell') has a very simple action to perform – one of Choice. The choice is between accepting the recommended action ('Yes' or 'Make it so'), or rejecting it (No), or Wait (for my decision).

ALTERED STATES OF CONSCIOUSNESS

William Johnston

William James

R.C. Zoehner

ANIMA/ANIMUS

In the Jung-Plato paradigm, three major strands of thought, pertaining to gender, come together. Plato's notion of an elective or eclectic affinity as 'the other half of one's soul' can be seen as Yin and Yang operating in the physical universe on individual beings in that capacity; and Jung's Anima/Animus – hitherto shrouded in mystery and 'etheriality' – can be seen as a _real_ guide to future actions.

From the Jungian perspective, Yolande Jacobi, Marie-Louise von Franz, and Timothy O'Neill, have each shown accord with particle physics and with Hinduism. They present vastly differing views and descriptions of the important construct, the Animus/Anima.

The two ladies, in _Man and his Symbols_, represent the 'A/A' in terms of the traditional concept of it being constructed to serve as a guide. It is formed by the collection and accumulation, _over countless aeons._ of individual characteristics of _real women_, so as to provide a _real picture_ of an entirely _fictive woman_ which, having served its purpose, becomes _entirely disposable._

Timothy O'Neill (as I understand him) offers, to the contrary, _nothing fictive._ Completely consistent with both Platonism and Hinduism, he gives us the A/A as a _real_ entity giving guidance towards union with a _real, unique,_ equal and opposite _pole_ of a higher-order entity.

O'Neill's attribution of equality and oppositeness follows the principles of Yin and Yang but the ladies do not even observe the placement of the two principles in regard of each other – which has considerable significance   (see YIN-YANG) and they base their treatment on the Mandala.

Experience is written into this very creditable rendering of the A/A from neurophysiology, psychology and philosophy by the input from Ethel Spector Person, Rollo May, C.S. Sherrington, Otto Rank, Janet and Freud, J.B. Priestley, Hinduism, the Sufi poets (and others), Christian apologist C.S. Lewis, St. Teresa of Avila, and so on. The list is endless, and includes the 'man in the street'.

ANTHROPIC PERSPECTIVE

David Peat outlines the Anthropic perspective very neatly for us. The universe that we know, says he, is formed by 'the great energy of the ten-dimensional superstring theory' of which we are aware only through ' very fine energy probes (light, X-rays, sound) involving energies that are negligible compared with those of the vast energies of superstrings and 'grand unification'.

The great energies of the superstrings are somehow shaped and formed by processes at a vanishingly small level. These processes are of such complexity and subtlety that they create elementary particles. If there are more massive particles around, then we simply cannot 'see' them (296).

Another important point that he makes is that Nature involves a *whole series of hierarchies* and that some scientists aver that *new levels of complexity are emergent structures* not to be expected on the basis of an underlying level. He dismisses this idea (p. 295) remarking that such ideas always suffer the defects of reductionism – exactly the same as remarked by Popper in *The Self and Its Brain*.

In short, all the physics we have ever studied, our own lives, and our consciousness are really enormously *fine corrections* to an underlying level. Our consciousness involves fine-tuned chemical and electrical processes that are negligible compared with those of the next level down the hierarchy of the Great Chain of Being. See Axis of Scale; Hinduism; etc.

ATTENTION

Like Awareness, Attention is multi-levelled. The 'operating system' of the brain/mind(Ego), i.e. the lowest parts of the brain (brain stem, limbic system, etc.), extending laterally below the mammalian and human brains to form the Triune brain, has a very different depth of interest from the User system at, or 'above', the highest level.

This can be seen vividly in *The Self and Its Brain* by Popper and Eccles. For example, in that work we have the self-conscious mind as

'Some multiple scanning and probing device that reads out from and selects from the immense and diverse patterns of activity in the cerebral cortex and integrates these selected components , so organizing them into conscious experience' (p. 363).

And the 'neuronal machinery' as

'A multiplex of radiating and receiving structures' (p. 362).

The point being made by the authors is that 'the experienced unity comes, not from a neurophysiological synthesis but from the proposed integrating character of the self-conscious mind. But, there are plenty of factors indicating that they are referring *only* to the procedures of the operating system as organized by the 'agent' (MacKay), aka 'Self 1' (Priestley).

The *'User'*, aka 'Self 2' (Priestley) or 'the determinator' (MacKay) determines the way ahead from the integrated 'picture' prepared for itself by the integration processes (as described by Mackay) from the brain's *neuronal machinery,* i.e. The Reptilian, the Mammalian, and the Human brains.

Popper and Eccles neglect, also, the brain's 'principle of convergence' which makes selection of the preferred action alternative by Sherrington's 'ultimate pontifical nerve-cell' comparatively simple. However, we are still faced with the task of identifying and locating the Priestley Self 3 which gives the nod, so to speak, to Self 2. (For more on Level see *Holography*).

AWARENESS

Awareness runs parallel to *Plurality of Consciousness* and to *Attention*, but there is yet another *perspective* on it that is presented by Roger Penrose, who remarks that great minds, poets, artists, composers, scientists, and Plato (he lists a dozen or so), seem to have a faculty of 'smelling out' truth and beauty that is more powerful than is given to most of us (SoM, 1995, p. 420).

He describes this faculty as a 'gift' for perceiving truth and beauty – Plato's 'the Good' – but it is possible that the faculty is a localized ability within a more general feeling of 'well-being and togetherness' pertaining to all living creatures even down to protozoa.

Although he ascribes the gift to the understandings of genius, he does point out that a unity with the works of Nature is potentially present in all of our *conscious brains*, which are woven from 'subtle physical ingredients' that enable us to perceive and make use of the *profound organization of our mathematically underpinned universe* which operates at many different levels.

However, any apparent disparity between his argument and mine is assuaged by his introduction of a protozoan – a paramecium – into considerations. Anyone who has engaged in microscopy is likely to prefer these endearing little creatures to something like an amoeba.

AXIS OF SCALE

The versatility, utility, and value of the Logistic growth function enable the use of an Axis of Scale which possesses similar properties. If this axis is taken as the abscissa (with orders of magnitude as its units), then 'p' (in the logistic) changes from a probability to a proportion. Better still, the ordinate can be seen as 'log (odds)', i.e. Good's measure of *plausibility*

However, the *Probability* from which the odds are determined is, in Bayesian theory, a conditional probability derived from (a) the probability of an event happening under stated conditions multiplied by (b) the likelihood of those conditions obtaining.

More properly it is the *sum* of all such likelihoods divided by a factor which sets the range of values obtained between zero and one.

Whole rafts and classes of sub-functions subsist under this arrangement, and there is a great similarity to the myriads of possibilities subsisting under the theory of 'strings', in particle physics, which introduce all kinds of problems stemming from infinities. But, thanks to Cantor, we know that infinities are structured and ordered (under the general heading, loosely, of the Transfinite).

This means that, within mathematical Platonism and von Bertalanffy's logico-mathematical regime, both the position and momentum of elementary particles *can* be determined. This supports the contention of John Polkinghorne that elementary particles are real.

His Christian apology is founded upon Platonism, and there are only two departures from it. The first is that his view does not assign a priority to the mental over the material, and this presents no problem to us because we know now that (under Comprehensive Reality) the whole *organism* subsumes both *the Agent* and *the Determinator,* (under an Ideal Form*)*.

The second difference is that Polkinghorne's perspective posits that the noetic world 'does not stand alongside God on equal terms but it depends upon him' (1988, p.77). In this respect, we have to remember that Polkinghorne by noetic means 'spiritual' in other contexts. Digging deeper, we find in one place that God holds everything together moment –to- moment and, in another place, God is content, by and large, to *allow* existence to go on (p. 58).

The essential feature, from a systems viewpoint, is that the Christian religion posits that God is outside (and above) Existence (p. 80). We can, therefore, conceive of God as a *User* of the physical universe; and Donald MacKay has God as an Author in 'dialogue' with his created 'stories' to influence and affect the whole 'Story'. This seems a radical difference from John Polkinghorne, and one which is more consonant with the notion of a wave of excitation sweeping through a network.

Regarding input to the physical universe system, this is easily accommodated by mathematical topography's variety of 'spaces'. For example, 'de Sitter space' and 'anti-de Sitter space' come to mind (see Paul Davies; Roger Penrose) in relation to hyperboloids. All kinds of twists, knots, manifolds, etc., are available in eminently respectable text-books.

However, returning to the Axis of Scale and to Cantor, systems theory finds the Logistic function even more valuable today than when it was praised by Ludwig von Bertalanffy nearly fifty years ago. This is because it seems to be applicable to the growth of information, per se, independent of context. If this is so, then it would truly be one of Matterssich's 'norms of nature'.

As such, it would provide a vast, real, network of overarching asymptotic curves into mathematical space which lead by definition into the Infinite and transfinite, and originate from various segments of the axis – which is exactly what we find. The line segments would cover the trajectories of the curves according to an infinite set of parameters, and it occurs naturally to the statistician that the principle of Maximum Likelihood might be applicable (see also the Appendix).

For the record, and for what it is worth, Mattessich's 'Ontological Assumption' of the Information Principle (pp. 314-5) reads: The *norms incorporated* in a system become *a fixed source* of information for this system, whereas the norms *temporarily imposed* upon the system by the environment constitute *a variable information source* for this system. Such information determines the characteristics and the behaviour of the system

It is noteworthy that von Bertalanffy pays more attention to categorization of *types* or *kinds* of information, such as *emotional, experiential, situational, etc.,* which offers more practical and mechanistic recognition for isomorphism.

It is not uncommon for those using mathematics to work in logarithms because of the immensity of the numbers involved. I have in mind people such as cosmologists, mathematicians, and philosophers, and the thought does not escape me that the measures of Subjective Probability, relating to *plausibility* rather than probability, are logarithmic. [Plausibility is 'Log odds']

Karl Popper discusses the declension – atoms, subatomic particles, sub-subatomic particles – in reference to the inadequacy of Reductionism – and to the 'Programme of Reductionism'. The particles are seen as being *real* (Polkinghorne), and along an Axis of Scale they can be separated out into zones or realms. For example, particle physicists give us the declension, in decreasing order of size, atoms, Fermions and Bosons, quarks and leptons, all, of course, within the volume of space-time which we experience 'normally'.

In these zones or realms there are to be seen parallels with the material plane, the lower astral plane, the higher astral plane, and the *causal plane* of Hinduism. Causality *seems* to be the same - in the interaction of light with matter and the exchange of photons, both at the 'causal level'.

In going 'deeper', i.e. further along the axis towards the infinite and transfinite, we enter the esoteric quantum field theory, supersymmetry, and string theory, etc., and become *transcendent*. In short, we enter (in the terms of Hinduism) the level of divinity in which YIN AND YANG co-operate *within* the entity.

There seems no scientific reason for denying this. We have facts, such as non-locality, speeds faster than light (rotational speeds?), the transfinite, set theory, the work of Godel, hidden dimensions, *and* we have the *need* for siting, somewhere, the mechanisms for ESP, such as Telepathy and Precognition (see *Hidden Dimensions; Higgs boson*)

BODY OF BELIEFS

I.J. Good, in *Probability and the Weighing of Evidence*, makes the point that any calculus of probability should (must) be founded upon a 'sound' body of beliefs. It is customary to look for qualities, such as coherence and consistency, and subjective probability is important because it affords *quantitative* weights of evidence to be accumulated in the calculus of *Likelihood* under those conditions.

'Jack' Good offered an example of short term weather forecasting so as to evaluate the likelihood of rain in the forthcoming few hours. Based on *evidence* for the proposition that it will rain during that time, he would decide whether or not to take an umbrella with him on a proposed sortie.

However, the usefulness of subjective probability is much greater than this. It has been used successfully and widely, for example, in the application of Jung's modes of Judgment and Perception (broken down into his four functions of sensation, feeling, intuition, and thinking) to Radar Probability Theory, Underwater Physiology, and countless other applications by use of the Logistic Growth Function.

In that function, the 'growth' is of information; and one particular benefit from plotting a curve of the function is that it can be broken down into sections covering periods of time. Whole 'families' of derived curves can also be generated from regular increases in a constant or someother parameter. This might be of particular interest to mathematicians such as Roger Penrose and Rudy Rucker.

Equally important is the fact that numerical weightings can be attached to linguistic 'signs', mostly words, according to the context in which they assume significance according to any particular theme. Human situation appraisal can be assessed, therefore, by machine if the value weightings are available for each word (sign) according to context and theme.

This is of huge potential for psycholinguistic analysis as well as for evolutionary psychology, because the individual word weightings will have been determined by heuristic learning. This principle, tested experimentally, gives promise also of being applicable to different stages of brain evolution. Human situation appraisal at the reptilian level has already been modelled successfully. See Bibliography.

BOUNDARIES

CARRYING OVER [from Logistic]

CATEGORISATION

It can be argued that correct categorisation – in one form or another - is vital to the continuance of all forms of life. A prime example is that both mathematical set theory and biological heuristic learning are based upon Categorisation. And, for that matter, so are religious Discernment and Escape from the predatory clutches of the social Leviathan.

In ordinary daily life we depend upon it, and the study of signs (in Semiotics) relates to *Meaning* in communications between individuals – both human and lower animals down to worms. Elizabeth Bates shows that the very same words can have different meanings according their contexts. But we don't need to be told that – we know from experience that different tones and gestures convey different meanings. [This matters desperately to lovers]

CAUSALITY [de Sitter Space]

CENTRAL ORDER

W.H. Thorpe, the celebrated ethologist, entitled one of his works, *Purpose in a World of Chance*, and this seems adequately to reflect one aspect of Man's predicament as a reflective animal. William Thorpe, himself reflects that he is, so to speak, 'a pragmatic dualist' (p. 113) but that the only kind of monism that he can envisage as being sensible is 'one of the Whiteheadian type'.

Thorpe's opinion is that which is often aired by process philosophers, namely that they are brought by their studies to conclude that some kind of theism is inevitable (p. 116). He cites Werner Heisenberg on this

The problem of values is nothing but the problem of our acts, goals and morals. It concerns the compass by which we must steer our ship if we are to set a true course through our life....I have a clear impression that all such [religious] formulations try to express man's relatedness to a central order. In the final analysis the central order, or the One...must win out.

William Thorpe believes that Heisenberg is 'entirely right' over this; and it seems likely that the viewpoint is one of many that all point to the same conclusion. Heisenberg goes on to remark the without this central order (i.e. 'the ethical norms of Christianity') terrible things may happen to Mankind, far more terrible even than 'concentration camps and atom bombs'.

That belief is more profound than it is in Jung's comments in similar vein, and it relates to a number of other issues. In particular, one such issue is the invitation (almost) to posit an equal and opposite 'central order' - an issue into which Jung delved unsuccessfully. The matter raises the question of whether there is one supreme 'orchestrator' of the social Leviathan's activities. C.S. Lewis was inclined to think that there is such an entity.

Rudy Rucker, in contradistinction to William Thorpe's 'pragmatic' dualism, expresses the 'desire' for it. He remarks that it would be nice if Cantor's 'two-substance' theory were true, because then we could have the mind or 'astral body' made up of some higher-level substance quite different from matter. As his book was published in 1982 he was clearly unaware of the relevant phenomena of Buddhism, Hinduism, and Mysticism.

Rucker may have been surprisingly near the mark in his semi-serious whimsical remark that we may have ectoplasmic souls, each made of Aleph-one aether-monads! He wrote:

It is hard to imagine ever observing such nested infinitesimals, but some useful theory, with observable consequences, may find its theoretical foundations in Absolutely Continuous Space. Or it could be that particles can be viewed as singularities of varying transfinite order. (p. 90).

Against this kind of background, it does not seem fanciful to wonder if the central order of 'the Good' may be multi-facetted and open to approaches from other quarters - such as from mathematical viewpoints. In the context of Evidence, this would take us straight away to Irving John Good's statistical 'landmarks' of *Plausibility* and of the quantizing the value of propositions.

In fact, it might be said that another 'landmark' was reached, shortly after Good's effort, which took the weighing of evidence literally into another dimension – the dimension of Scale posted by Rudy Rucker. This happened when it was discovered (independently) that *Plausibility*, i.e. 'log(odds)', is derivable from the well-known growth function, i.e. the *Logistic* function.

For example, plotting along an axis of scale in the conventional units of 'powers of ten' or 'orders of magnitude', the magnitude of growth over periods of time (in many areas) shows up as a typical asymptotic curve. This takes one into Infinite regions because the final value of the function can be reached only at infinity.

Jack Good brought personal *subjective opinion* into the various realms of information theory, decision-making (praxeology) which theretofore had been austerely inflexible and based upon the notion of *perfection*, i.e. perfect coins, perfect dice, etc., which were unreal. The price to be paid for this benefit is that personal subjective opinion actually *introduces* error (in the statistical sense).

He had anticipated this, however, by insisting that any 'calculus of probability' utilizing his measures must be based upon sound foundations, such as the customary qualities of coherence, consistency, and (from Popper) testability. Clearly, not every idea or hypothesis is open to testing, but its 'degree of isomorphism' with a standard model (say, mathematics) would do.

However, even the most hardened sceptic – approaching the fanatical – would deny that the notion of treating words as Peircean *signs* and assigning *numerical weights to each word for a range of contexts and themes* improves decision making and gives it, so to speak, a sharper edge.

The siting of Werner Heisenberg's *values* in our acts, goals, and morals in *the One* certainly allows each individual a *choice* – such as 'to follow or not to follow'. And, even if we allow mathematical Platonism to obtain, together with Donald MacKay's mechanistic embodiment, the issue of that bi-polar choice remains.

The crux of this matter, it seems, is that the individuality of Good's landmark notion can be reasonably extended, *in principle*, to relate to Groups of individuals provided that they can agree upon the meaning of any proposition. This may be regarded as a tall order, but it should be possible to find agreement within agreed definitions (perhaps by using the Central Limit Theorem).

This having been said, one can foresee the potential for setting the customary confidence limits for the credibility of any natural language proposition. For example, as I have just mentioned, the Central Limit Theorem of Statistics posits that the mean of a number of means remains the same whatever the sampling, and this would some arrangement of a central order.

Be this as it may, the crux of the Jung-Plato paradigm is centred upon a notion savouring of 'Exactness in a World of Apparent Chance' (pace William Thorpe). Exactitude comes from both Jung and from Plato. From the latter we have the notion of two different parts of a soul seeking eventual re-union and, consequently, uplift into a higher spiritual Realm.

From Jung, we start from the fact (a) that there is sufficient isomorphism to justify (i) the encephalized mind(Ego) and (ii) to posit a world of only relationships and fields. Additionally, we end up having the capital concept of the Anima/Animus being a *real* guide to its other part, namely the Elective or Eclectic Affinity – no wonder Jung was so attracted to the notion !

CLAIRVOYANCE

Even in a most esteemed dictionary of philosophy the term 'Clairvoyance' is booted into the long grass (to use a sporting metaphor) and is replace by the term 'Paranormal'. An ordinary English dictionary defines Clairvoyance as 'The power of discerning things beyond the normal range of sense or perception', which seems adequate.

There are those who would prefer the latter to the former because it contains fewer 'metaphysical assertions'. Others might prefer the account given by J.B. Priestley in *Man and Time* because it relates to everyday *living experience* and to metaphysical assertions which are geared to *practicality* and to *mathematical expression*, i.e. Time dimensionality.

Clairvoyance or 'the Parnormal' is, however, often taken to include Telepathy, Psychokinesis, Precognition, and Survival after bodily death. There is no definition, in the dictionary of philosophy, of 'Mind' – only items under 'the philosophy of mind' and the mind-body problem'.

It is illuminating that within the forty-one lines of text covering those two items there is not a single mention of *brain* Is this not carrying academic caution too far? The question is rhetorical – but it *does* make a fair point. However, clear-cut, testable, definitions can now be given – thanks to systems technology.

Systems technology is one of three branches of Systems Theory listed by Ludwig von Bertalanffy. He gave these branches as *systems science, systems technology,* and *systems philosophy*; and Richard Mattessich added *systems methodology*. However, the real breakthrough comes through reference to computer *systems*. [The italics emphasize the need to consider not just computers but the systems in which they are embedded but also the '*Users*' which they serve]

CLINICAL TOOLS

The committal of Personality to the brain/mind(Ego), together with the   close isomorphism between the brain's 'mental system' and a real-time computer system, make *personality assessment* both more understandable and easier to execute.

For example, back in the 1980s, when the isomorphism was announced, it was considered that methods of studying personal concepts offered no way of being useful other than ideographically. For example, Philip Vernon (p. 21) remarked that Osgood's Semantic Differential, the 'Q-sort, and G. Kelly's 'Reptest', offered only 'constructs about people, not about jobs, goals, etc'.

The application of Pierce's notions of words as indexes to meanings, as they were described in Elizabeth Blakes, *Language and Context*, led to experiments in *Linguistic Analysis* by attaching numerical weights to words per person or computer program, which could be summed to give an indication of value as pointers to particular contexts in regard of particular themes. [It was said at the time that this provided theoretical foundations for Kelly's Personal Construct Theory]

In my report of the successful experiment, a range of prospective and potential examples is given to illustrate computer usage in this respect. It was acknowledged, also, at the time that this notion was original, and some correspondence to this effect ensued.

COHOMOLOGY

David Peat remarks that nature may be unchanged by certain transformations of structures in a fundamental space. He is writing about 'superstring space' and the possibility of 'recovering' certain laws by relating such structures to something like Penrose's twistor approach whereby they prove to be more fundamental than 'the action principles that have been traditionally used in both classical and quantum physics (p. 334).

Not only is this an example of 'thinking before acting', but it ties in with such things as 'world lines' and smacks of an epitheoretical viewpoint. Cohomology is difficult to describe.   It is non-local and involves the 'gluing' together of 'patches' in differing manifolds in twistor theory.

Roger Penrose opines that sheaf cohomology is 'an excellent example of a Platonic notion where, like the system of complex numbers, it seems to have a life of its own "going far beyond any particular way in which one may choose to represent it" ' (2004, p. 992)

COMMAND

Ruth Munroe saw herself as the 'I' of common parlance – she had Freudian inclinations, so (loosely) she equated herself with the biological Ego-function. Gordon Rattray Taylor remarked 'I am me' and thought largely of brain/mind functions. And, Danah Zohar declared 'I am my relationships'. Each of them presented an incomplete picture and misrepresented the Truth (in my opinion).

Closer to the Truth is Jung's notion that Ego-consciousness is governed by some superordinate entity which is not in its 'mind-set'. He was wrong, however, to place 'Ego-consciousness' in his non-material psyche. See *Strong Dualistic Hypothesis*. Closest to the Truth is Sherrington's notion of brain and 'psyche' collaborating separately but being joined at a higher level as part of a higher system.

In that case, the Command fiat identified by William James emanates from a 'Spirit Body' manifesting itself through the Causal zone (see Hinduism), and we can perceive something akin to that in the *Strong Dualistic Hypothesis* advanced by Popper and Eccles – but, like Jung, they are wildly wrong in their understanding of the Users of computers and their placement of authority.

Unfortunately, we cannot escape this question of Command – some Jungians claim that Jung avoided the issue. Even the hardest notions of determinacy are faced with the fact that unless the individual has *at least* the freedom to be *different* from what appears to be its allotted course the individual is nothing but an automaton acting out its *story*.

The modification of Jungian theory, i.e. the encephalized mind(Ego), boosts the concept of a *psychagogue* which is, in fact, one's Animus/Anima acting out its role as a Guide. But, of course, in view of mathematical Platonism and *Comprehensive Reality*, it is operating from knowledge of its Goal, held at a higher level, and moved by concepts of Mysticism (Indwelling, Union, and merger (see William Johnston).

COMMAND FIAT

Jung asserts that anyone wishing to have an answer to the problem of evil (which he sees as determinant reality) has need, first and foremost, of *self-knowledge*. This knowledge is inclusive of one's *potential* for each and every <u>kind</u> of evil, and it poses the need for avoiding illusion (p. 305). [It also conflicts with his statement that we cannot imagine evil]

More generally, one can see from this that, as well as self-knowledge, there is a need of *discernment* and a need of *commitment* This brings us, again, face-to-face with Sherrington's ultimate pontifical nerve-cell, which may be, or may not be, putative. [I have in mind MacKay's mechanistic embodiment of a formula]

Unless the organism is a complete automaton there must be somewhere a system that gives the Command fiat.   William James makes explicit reference to the fiat, as does Rollo May.   And, this brings one to the thoughts of Rollo May (existentialist) and of Otto Rank (as described by Ruth Munroe as a psychotherapist), each of whom features the WILL.

Rollo May (p. 243) refers to James's, fiat, 'Let it be so' and, on the same page, makes the point that one refers to oneself in saying, 'I will make it so'.   Importantly, he introduces the concept of 'the realization of potential', which is *the* essential feature of computers and, also, one of Aristotle's four types of causality (as seen by Joan Wynn Reeves on p. 41).

The sequence presented by Rollo May, on the same page, is the Command sequence of human experience 'I conceive-I can-I will-I am'.   On page 202, Rollo May defines man's task as being:...to unite love and will. They are not united by automatic biological growth but must be part of our development'.

Otto Rank makes very similar points.

COMMON SENSE

In general, 'common sense' is one of the most widely understood yet most indefinable terms used in the English Language. Its precise meaning is dependent upon the nature, nurture, and circumstances of the individual using it. And, the faculty of applying common sense may extend back down the evolutionary trail as far as Protozoa.

The notion of common sense carries with it, also, a necessity to select the appropriate words when trying to define it, but the difficulty, too, of finding *any* such word (Lexicographers tell us, in any case, that definitions at base are inevitably circular). See Body of Beliefs.

If we consider only human and artificial 'intelligence' we are 'stumped' *ab initio* for two reasons. The first is that 'intelligence' has a number of different meanings.   The second is that any selected reason is inadequate and, at best, incomplete. See Taxonomy and Personality.

These limitations put us at a disadvantage in communicating with each other (for person *and machine)* but they place us in very *dangerous* situations when facing our enemies. Sherrington, for example, delineates man's enemies as Nature, Man, and Man Himself, i.e. each individual's 'inner self'. See Warship Analogy, Personality, Encephalized Mind(Ego), social Leviathan.

Likewise, we are faced with problems in dealing with and expressing our emotions, which are linked with heuristic learning all along the evolutionary trail. Poetry is useful in this, rather than natural language, and this is generally acknowledge by scientist and layman, alike. See the Appendix.

The Platonic 'take' on this is that strong emotions, such as Love, Truth, Beauty, Justice, Mercy, etc., are the Good (which should be followed) and that their opposites, such as Hate, Falsehoods, Ugliness, Injustice, 'economies with the Truth' and so on, should be avoided or controlled. The consequences of any such Badness, for Plato, are Metempsychosis; and this is supported by the models offered by the Warship Analogy. See Process, Process Image/ Ideal Form, Metempsychosis.

It might appear that common sense flies out of the window when one is faced with the social Leviathan (politicians, administrators, religiosos, etc.) or with strong emotions (Love, Hate, etc.), injustices, infelicities, and other all too human frailties. But primitive mam (when the social Leviathan was in its infancy) was equally frail.

Jung, echoing the Delphic oracle, asserted the prime axiom and injunction, 'Know Thyself', but, Jung, himself, seems unable to do this. Without going deeply into his private life, we can see this in '*Memories, Dreams, Reflections*' by his assurance, for example, that he knew better than Freud about his own dreams and in talks with his psychagogues.

Again, we might think that computers can do it for us (i.e. applying common sense), but that has its difficulties for computers have to be programmed and science-fiction stories about self-developing computers and the dangers they might pose are abundant.   Subjective Probability, coupled with our existing massively powerful computers might, in principle, provide us with Truth (limited to certain Perspectives). See Perspectivism (von Bertalanffy).

Jung's particular individual contributions to Science are often under-rated and misunderstood in equal measure.   And, he did everyone a disservice by differentiating only between Consciousness and 'the Unconscious'. This seems to savour of his desire to get away from Freud.

In particular, 'common sense' should have told him that if the *subconscious* provided by Janet and by Freud is a sound idea, and likewise ideas of a *superconscious* come in from several quarters, then the collective term *Unconscious* is not particularly useful (unless it be qualified further).

For example, we know from computer analogies that 'consciousness' is usually accompanied by activities which are not in our conscious minds but operate specifically for (and during) activities in *real-time*.   It would be common sense to call these computer–like processes by the name of 'periconscious'. This would then include the psychological 'specious present' and the mathematical 'twistor'.

Singularly useful is 'The Axis of Scale', which is commonly used (in slightly differing formats) by scientists, philosophers, and mathematicians. This fills the gap, so to speak, between the physical universe and structured forms of Infinity and the Transfinite. It allows new discoveries to be slotted in. See 'Axis of Scale'.

Another notable feature is the gradual 'formalizing' of common sense through, in order, Aristotle, Bacon, Ouspensky, and Good. The escalation in the ways of the so-called 'noetic acquisition of knowledge' ranges from Aristotle's deductive logic and Bacon's inductive logic to the mysticism inherent in Ouspensky's intuitive logic and the direct and simultaneous acquisition of knowledge from the experience of Others. See Quartic Organum.

114

I. J. Good devised measures of awarding numerical values to propositions in natural language. He used Likelihood rather than Probability by using the logarithms of 'betting odds', and those measures were subsequently keyed into Information Theory by way of a common growth function called the Logistic function. This was done separately and independently from Good's work to fulfil the utilitarian necessity arising in Radar Probability Theory.

It is not difficult to perceive from the above that 'common sense' in humans is basically a derivative expansion – together with the expanding brain of an organism of unknown dimensions. A popular number (for the dimensions) is eleven, but Rudy Rucker write of 'Infinite–dimensional' organisms.

Similarly, the higher animals appear to possess, on occasions, qualities which to human eyes are deontic and/or normative. An example would be a blue-tit fluttering desperately (?) to fly through a glass window calmly hopping immediately on to a stick offered by a human being and allowing itself to be transported through a house to fly off Immediately on reaching the outside.

Another example would be that of a cat launching itself furiously at a dog which appeared (?) to be threatening a small baby lying in its carry-cot on the ground – and such examples abound.

To sum up, then, we can conjecture that common sense is a composite ability to comprehend situations from the point of view of actions in ways other than intellectual ability. The functions comprising this capacity come from different parts of the brain – ranging from the brain stem to the prefrontal areas. As a consequence of this each person varies in his/her degree and nature of common sense; in principle each person has a common sense 'profile'.

In a way, these characteristics are reflected in slang which offers a kind of spectrum stretching from 'brightness' to 'dimness' without disapprobation. Where the person does not in any way follow a sensible course of action because of wilfulness, or waywardness, or to show defiance (at stupid cost to themselves), or petty childishness, etc., the slang term 'thick' is more appropriate.

Examples abound and we can all recall observing friends, colleagues, family members, bystanders, etc., being 'thick'. Most of us can remember ourselves 'being thick'. But it is one thing to admit it, and quite another thing to be called it. So tact and discretion are required always, *and good will*. If we know someone who is thick of choice, apparently, then they are 'prayer jobs', i.e. beyond help except for that last resort. See, also, *Sex and Love*.

COMPREHENSIVE REALITY

This is the scheme advanced by Donald MacKay of 'mechanistic embodiment' based on his knowledge of real-time systems for Information Processing and Communication (with Others).

COMPUTER SYSTEM

CONSCIOUNESS

In terms of unitary consciousness, Danah Zohar views 'consciousness as relationships' (p. 82). It is probable that the term used by Taylor, i.e. 'plurality of consciousness', is more appropriate (or even the 'levels of awareness' used by many. The terms are theory-laden, and it might be best always to identify the appropriate context and referential theme.

Her claim that consciousness is at the 'primary level of existence' may raise a few eyebrows, and beg suggestions that 'existence' might be replaced, say, by 'experience', or some other word. But, more difficult to accept is her assertion that 'consciousness is a pattern of relationship' that is the 'wave side' of wave particle duality.

This statement implies a massive amount of organization that is not reflected in her description of the utility of bosons. In contradistinction, the organization behind the 'Hindu yogic tradition' or, more broadly the 'Sino-Asiatic model', is exactly what one would expect. It is notable that such models were devised by five thousand years of *deep thought*' (boosted by experience). Also that Jung misused them.

CONTEXTS AND THEMES

In human thinking, there can be no absolute or certain meaning without a statement of the *context* of an event or a situation. One is guided towards the right context partly by one's personality, partly by one's linguistic knowledge and ability, partly by one's intentions, and partly by a number of other factors. In any case, the use of words in dictionaries, i.e. in Lexicology, is ultimately circular.

We sharpen up our thinking by considering words as *signs* or *indexes* (see Elizabeth Bates) to contexts, and I have shown experimentally that human thought can reproduce (seemingly) thought at the Reptilian level by treating words as signs in the judgement of Safety/Danger. I did this by using words as *weighted* signs in regard of contexts.

Even so, our thinking is geared also to our motivation at different priority levels for differing goals from different perspectives. And, according to our individual normative and deontic weightings, we establish some kind of 'priority ordering matrix' by algorithms relating our assessment of the probable outcome of some action in terms of utility in achieving some or all of our *goals*.

This, it seems, applies to all living things at or above the unicellular level, and to the most abstract and subtle human thinking. In the latter case, for example, I have long been slightly puzzled by the arrival of the number zero which, to me, seems the result of mental 'trickery' governed by utility.

Ludwig von Bertalanffy writes well on this. He points out that discursive thinking can never exhaust the infinite manifoldness of ultimate reality. Thus, he argues, the categories – the vital categories – of our experience and thinking appear to be determined by biological as well as cultural factors (1973, p. 261).

On the same page he writes that ultimate reality is a union of opposites. Any statement must be supplemented by antithetic statements. And, this very sensible requirement takes me back to the number zero which can only be derived from the existence of a category called a *set* (see Rudy Rucker).

COSMIC PAROCHIALISM

As far as is known, the term 'Cosmic Parochialism' is made public for the first time in this monograph. Yet, it seems appropriate for a notion that embraces so many 'perspectives' on Existence and, if accepted, would explain so much. It might be considered as a codicil to the Jung-Plato paradigm, or to the already accepted Sino-Asiatic paradigm.

It is pertinent to perspectives on Christian dogma and, therefore, to W.E.R. Mons and to C.G. Jung. And, the term fans out, so to speak, in its variety of applications – some of which overlap. At least five such fields come to mind immediately, and they are as follows and their explication helps to illustrate fully my meaning.

Poetry and Mysticism are represented in my list by William Blake in his references to Los's Halls. Literary applications abound in the fictional works of C.S. Lewis. Cosmic Parochialism also describes neatly the thoughts of William James (and others) concerning pluralism and polytheism in relation to the 'superconscious'.

The term relates, additionally to Plato's notion of Creation and the demiurgoi – as is admirably set out by Joan Wynn Reeves (in *Body and Mind in Western Thought*) – and these overlap with C.S. Lewis and with Jung, in particular. Needless to say, it fits in some ways with proper Science Fiction, and with some parts of Fantasy (the field of which is growing apace). And, it accommodates certain kinds of biological, cosmological and neurophysiological data and propositions that are steadily accumulating.

DATA AND REALITY

In the field of Information Technology, as in daily living generally, a fundamental distinction is made between data and Information. Data becomes information only when *more than one* datum have been analysed, interpreted, received or dispatched. In common parlance, the basic unit of data is called a 'bit' (i.e. binary digit).

A similar distinction is made by Whitehouse in his *Process Philosophy*. The minimal unit is an *event* which is called an *occasion of experience*, and which cannot exist on its own – there has two be more than one occasion of experience.

This fits very easily into the notion common to a number of different fields of *relationships* and information being prime features of, say, Existence. William Kent, for example, distinguishes between 'Data and *Reality*': he worked for *IBM* and his book was first published in 1978. It fits, also, with Donald MacKay's scheme of 'Comprehensive Reality' – featuring *mechanistic embodiment.*

More important thn these conjectures, however, is that Information, discussed in these terms is consonant with Set Theory and with the growth of a package of information from Zero (the empty set) to Transfinity. And, with Subjective Probability (Plausibility and Weight of Evidence) and the Logistic function – describing growth asymptotically. These provide a sound basis for very many 'norms of nature'.

All taken together, an excellent case seems to appear for mathematical Platonism and for models of Existence furnished by the Sino-Asiatic models and the Hindu yogic tradition. From this, an enhanced and expanded form of a *Semantic Web* may be fashioned as a general purpose *analytical tool.*

Be this as it may, one is drawn back to Science and mathematics as the roots of Reality, and, as John Polkinghorne asserts, leptons and quarks are *real* entities. So, coming back to the notion of a 'world' composed only of processes, and/or Information, and/or measurable units of Scale, etc., one finds oneself with the thoughts of Lee Smolin on these things. And, the Axis of Scale is a great help on such things.

It may seem rather strange that Smolin's thoughts lie in the very conjectural regions of 'quantum cosmology' (his term), but he mentions this in reference to a bound (the Beckenstein bound). This can be placed along the Axis of Scale, along with other interesting bounds, such as the Planck limits of Space and of Time. And this takes one into a whole new realm of conjecture and speculation in *psychiatry* – some 'nice' and some 'very nasty' (taking one into practices that are illogical, painful and injurious, and/or even illegal in some places.

Stopping short at this point, it can be said that the core of the debate is centred upon how Information can travel across 'bounds' on the axis of scale. In the physical universe this pertains to so-called 'singularities' (see Penrose; Rucker; Davies; Smolin; et al.

It is particularly noteworthy that some points of this kind, can be an order of magnitude in which the origin of information growth may start - as is visible along a logistic curve from which several other such curves may be 'spliced off' to cover, say, 'epochs'. (see also Cosmic Parochialism)

DECISION-MAKING and PRAXEOLOGY

'Praxeology is the science of decision-making'

DEMIURGOI

John Polkinghorne seems particularly upset by the concept of demiurgoi, yet he claims to differ from Plato in only two things – both of which are governed by his articles of faith. He really could be expected to find the notion of demiurgoi acceptable, because the notion is eminently plausible.

He attacks the notions, put forward by Paul Davies, of these demi-gods while being quite willing to accept 'angels' and a God who 'holds together moment-by-moment the 'entire immensity of Being'. Together with angels, Polkinghorne accepts the possibility of beings who 'are not rooted in the material'.

DIAGRAMMATIC REPRESENTATION

Systems theorists and particle physicists seem to be at each extreme end of polarized opinion over this subject. The former are, in my opinion, wildly over-enthusiastic about the power of 'isomorphism', and the latter find they can only communicate with each other by using diagrams which have nothing to do with actual phenomena.

My work in computers at one time led me into a region somewhere between the extremes and forced me to gain arcane knowledge that I could not use at the time but, much later, proved very useful. Through this, I found about needs to balance 'pure theory' with 'practical necessity'.

By this, I mean that some computer projects are so massive that they cannot be developed and built without imposing huge drains upon resources. I speak, therefore, from experience over this; but I'm sure a good number of project managers will agree with me about the importance of certain measures.

For example, I argued fiercely that 'program flowcharts' (*Maps*) should be accompanied by charts of individual 'process-flow' (*Itineraries* through the flowchart networks). However, when the leader of the contractors and I looked up – with some effort – the contract specification, we found that it specified that processes should _not_ be so described.

It is quite possible, I believe, that had the full cost of 'doing it properly' been disclosed to the appropriate authorities before contractual agreements were exchanged, then a deleterious political action might have been taken. On the other hand, the amounts of time and money wasted by documenters, repair engineers, Users, et al, were certainly not insignificant. The MoD team of documenters were very grateful for the information that I gave them.

The huge number of computer systems, world-wide, is rather alarming. However, 'trade-offs' _do_ have to be made, and I can reveal no more on such projects. I can express my sympathy with large commercial firms who, almost inevitably, face the problem of watching their ordering systems growing ever slower and unreliable and having to make policy decisions in this kind of background.

DIMENSIONS

There is a whole class of 'string' theories in regard of elementary particles and a quantum theory of gravity.   In many of them our universe is posited to contain extra dimensions curled up too tightly to be seen directly.   The simplest notion is of nine dimensions of which *six* are *compactified*.

Dimension of Time can be accommodated in mathematical theory – as can a dimension of Scale. An 'axis of scale' provides a measuring stick along which various bounds can be marked, such as Planck limits for Space and for Time.   Such a device is essential for reference to, say, orders of magnitude and extension into the physical universe's Environment.

DIMENSIONAL TIME

Ouspensky – Bennett => Analogous to Space

De Sitter Space - Hyperboloid Universe => Plato (in some ways)

DUALISM

(a) Dualism Types

(b) Dualism of Properties

At base-level this reduces to differences of such things as *Spin, Rotation, or Direction*.   For example, the natural unit of spin (supplied by quantum mechanics) is the natural numbers (i.e. Integers) for Bosons and for Fermions a spin of 1/2, 3/2, 5/2, etc. The 'Higgson' (Higgs boson) must have spin 0.   (Gell-Mann, p. 196).

Cited, also, by Murray Gell-Mann is the so-called 'Zipf's Law' devised in the early 1930s by George Kingsley Zipf.   This is one of the so-called scaling laws or power laws in the physical, biological, and behavioural sciences.   Gell-Mann places Zipf's law under empirical theory (p. 92) in terms of rank (as an abscissa).

However (without working it through) it seems highly likely to me that the association with rank can be dropped and the succession of rational numbers along an axis at regular unit intervals might be changed from a fraction with constant numerator 1 to a *proportion* derived from the previous number divided by the present number.

The logarithm of that proportional number could then be related to the Logistic measure of growth and the power law would be a part of formal Information Theory.   A number of my papers in the 1960s demonstrated the wide spread of applications of the Logistic functions – one of which related to particle physics, as I remember, and another which portrayed structured 'hidden' foundations for the Logistic..

In terms of spin, for example, the set of ordered natural numbers pertaining to bosons could be represented by the Logistic curve, whereas the set of rational numbers representing the fermions could not be so represented without an adjustment to the abscissa. This may just reflect that, under certain conditions, fermions may become bosons.

ENCEPHALIZED MIND(EGO)

ENGINE DRIVER (See, also, ATTENTION)

Jung, and Popper and Eccles, greatly underestimated the power, autonomy, and the general attributes and functions of the evolved human brain. The encephalization of the mind(Ego) largely solves that problem, but it does not *eradicate* the problem. Nor does it eliminate the problem of *Command* and the sender of the *Command Fiat*. The distinction between a programmer and a User illuminates this.

The User of the body/mind(Ego) does not need the exhaustive knowledge possessed by the designer and developer of the software, i.e. the programmer or rather the team of programmers. The User (i.e. the *Command element)* needs high-level knowledge of the system, of course, and a lifetime, almost, of developing it into an efficient operating entity; plus good documentation.

The point I am trying to make is that our knowledge of computers has grown so much, and so rapidly, since their advent (in the middle of the last century) that vessels and vehicles barely need Command elements. The concept from Natural Theology of an engine driver is about the best analogy that I can think of.

The comparison was made by Alister Hardy, in *The Biology of God* and, in my opinion, it is an excellent one for several reasons. It fits extremely well with Ouspensky's notion of *dimensional time,* and with Priestley's interpretation of it, and with Bennett's mathematical background of Priestley's constructs. Indirectly, therefore, it is consonant with Mysticism and ESP.

The Engine driver's lot is mostly that of Attentivity (and perhaps 'nipping out' of the cab to change points). And, round about that time (the advent of computers), the estimable Roger Delgado was presenting *experimental evidence* that a full-grown bull could be controlled in its movements by remote control sufficiently well to ensure safety for the operator in close proximity to the animal. [I have seen the video].

EPITHEORETICAL ANALYSIS

EVIDENCE

Judgment and Perception cannot proceed on the 'testability' of hypotheses alone. There are any number of hypotheses, for example, that call for faith, and Christianity is outstandingly commendable for establishing bodies of people to investigate the *evidence* for supporting faith with justified belief.

Apart from religion, however, there are numerous examples in Science of instances wherein testability is out of the question. In such cases, conjectures can be made and tested, but the circumstances of the application are so remote from the original hypothesis that they are of little value.

This is where subjective probability – as part of Information Theory – is of significant importance. In principle, every conceivable hypothesis can be awarded a numerical value and a weight of evidence accumulated that reflects the Likelihood being true. Thus, even infinitesimals can make a contribution to an overall numerical judgment. [Jung points out that in the categorization of Good and of Evil each represents a *judgment*] (p. 304).

It follows that in regard of Jung's more 'way out' assertions it may be a good policy to tie them down so far as possible to *facts*. As many of his visions and personifications are drawn from his personal experiences, it is desirable that any judgment of his reports should be from the judge's personal experience – thus showing that the phenomenon reported is possible, whatever the mechanism behind it.

I have such experience, of which the contents and the prevailing circumstances were also duly recorded. I have half-a-dozen such 'visionary' occasions in each of which there were events which are very, very unlikely to have occurred by chance and which indicate an outstandingly high degree of *Plausibility* for Clairvoyance.

Examples of these phenomena are given in the Appendix, and speaking professionally, as a Statistician, they are sufficient, contained in my personal Body of Beliefs, for me to set my life-style to accord with them.

It is not possible to give a definitive description of Evidence – such a provision has to be qualified, at least, by context and theme. For example, how can one be rigorous about over the matter of intuitive knowledge and perception – and yet equivalent functions are found in real-time computer systems. There are many instances of such isomorphism. Likewise, there are equivalents in music and in other forms of the presentation of information.

An everyday, pragmatic kind of example of 'Plausibility' is given by Good in his decision-making about the state of the weather during a proposed shopping expedition. His calculus of probabilities is based upon meteorological information, e.g. are the clouds heavy (nimbus) or light (cirrus), what is the nature of the wind, what is the direction of the wind, what is its strength, and so on.

We can gauge whether there is anything better than plausibility by reference to general purpose dictionaries, say, Chambers (CD) or the Shorter Oxford English Dictionary (SOED). We find, then, that everything said in the foregoing paragraphs is endorsed in the august pages of those excellent works.

Each dictionary breaks the word 'Evidence' into loosely the same seven contexts, one of which referring to proving or disproving a proposition. Jack Good, we might say, took it from there. And, the subsequent derivation of his measure from the logistic growth function accentuated its power and cemented it into more formal Information Theory – to be regarded, in particular, as the growth of *information* over sections of its range.

But, the growth of information applies to propositions in all the seven contexts, and each context has its own sets of *utilities* and their *values*, together with its own set of indexical signs (see Bates).   The elaboration of these squirrels down into vast, ordered and inter-linked, arrays of sets of dictionaries of contexts and themes.

Looking sideways, perhaps, and from a distance, we should see Rucker's 'nested infinitesimals'.   And, looking 'upwards' and from 'inside', we might even see his 'singularities'.

These are exactly what would be expected to emerge from the process of evolution using and developing heuristic searches and relational memories.   As the development of computer technology continues apace, so it exhibits layers of information processing, each with nodes and arranged in hierarchies.   It is not unreasonable to wonder if these also exist in the world of neural networks and/or in its foundation layers.

We come, therefore, to questions of *central order*. Accompanying these, there will be questions of utility and of evidence and value, and the huge benefit obtained therein by Good's discovery of *Plausibility*.   For example, the proposition of 'there will soon be rain' has a range of significances that is of far less consequence than the proposition of 'there is visible order in Evolution'

Jung, for instance, posited 'biological turmoil' and seemed to perceive little merit in genetics and heredity. But, the natural quarternion presents him with hard evidence which attracts immense weighting and is not disputatious.   There *is* order running throughout the whole of evolution.

EVIL

From experience and observation it does not seem difficult to categorize evil as 'determinant reality', as did Jung. It is more difficult to understand Jung's comment that 'in practical terms...good and evil are no longer so self-evident' (p. 304). [there appears to me an element of self-justification in his 'Late Thoughts' chapter]

Even more difficult to comprehend is his statement that 'We stand face to face with the terrible question of evil and we do not even know what is before us, let alone what to pit against it' (p. 305).   A major obstacle to comprehension of his words is his erroneous assertions about (i) personality, (ii) the psyche, and (iii) the goal of the psyche.

A much more appropriate question is as to whether evil is orchestrated overall by some malignant entity. C.S, Lewis may be a useful author to consult for two reasons. First that he wrote the two works on 'Screwtape' (a minor devil), namely *The Screwtape Letters* and *Screwtape Proposes a Toast*.   The second reason is that his science fantasy trilogy, especially *That Hideous Strength*, is very reflective of today's society, even seventy years after it was written. C.S. Lewis was 'inclined to believe in an arch-devil'

Logically, it seems today that all the evil obtaining in the world is being orchestrated by some power or principle. It is even the first of Mattessich's five ontological assumptions, i.e. the 'Principle of Polarity' (p. 307). This reads:

Being (i.e. any kind of existing entity) presupposes another 'being' of opposite polarity. This results in a tension, the release of which tends to annihilate (fully or partly) one or both of these entities, or to create a new one with its own opposite.

Mattessich continues, to reflect that one might even regard the polarity principle, together with the periodicity principle, as 'the key to the phenomenon of existence'. This is pretty daunting stuff, and it is difficult to believe that anyone who is (apparently) devoid of so much necessary knowledge could utter it.

Even as a 'sounding board' Mattessich's five ontological assumptions do not seem to carry cogency that comes anywhere near to that of Whitehead or, for that matter, von Bertalanffy.

FREE WILL

Roger Penrose 'tentatively' suggests that 'consciousness' may be some manifestation of a 'quantum-entangled internal cytoskeletal state' and its involvement in the interplay between quantum and classical levels of activity (SoM, p. 376). His idea is that our neural networks are continually influenced by cytoskeletal activity as a manifestation of 'Free Will'.

Penrose advances the dualistic idea in an attempt to explore how such influence could be effected at a scale much larger than single quantum particles (p. 350). The idea is plausible, but it must be weighed against other *factual* phenomena such as Sherrington's *principle of convergence* exhibited by the brain so as to ease the performance of the 'single ultimate pontifical cell'. There seems no good reason for this 'cell' being a non-local affect. [He is sympathetic to Danah Zohar's ideas]

On the other hand, Hiroshi Motoyama points out what any machine-code programmer knows, i.e. that the difference between one bit being set or cleared in a program can have an enormous effect. Roger Penrose's conception of neuron's having the role of a *magnifying device* is rather similar to the notions of Popper and Eccles expressed in *The Self and Its Brain* – except that it is in reverse.

Their concept is of 'some multiple scanning and probing device that reads out from and selects from the immense and diverse patterns of activity in the cerebral cortex and integrates these selected components, so organizing them into the unity of conscious experience' (p. 363). Surely the two notions can be brought together in some way (?!).

There are, in fact, several ways of accommodating the two notions – but not under unitary consciousness. For example, and without venturing into religious territory, we can distinguish between the awareness, or the noesis, of differing subsystems of one entity.

And, the entity, itself, can be a spirit body (within and outside the physical universe) with its Life Force being broken into yin and yang principle co-operating with each other in 'manifestations' of men and women.   After all, Roger Penrose, himself, admitted to dualism.

Moreover, in Donald MacKay's 'mechanistic embodiment' and/or mathematical Platonism, there is always the option of doing something different from what is prescribed. Otherwise, the organism is nothing but an automaton.

FREUDIAN THEORY

Freud built upon the work of Janet to formulate his notions of the *'subconscious'* and the *'conscious'* mind.   His constructs, such as the *instincts*, the *id*, the *Ego*, and the *Superego*, are well enough known, but it may not be so well known that he saw also a 'conscience' and that these entities were entirely fictive.

Thus, Freud's theories are consonant with most aspects of evolutionary psychology and with other theories which suppose mysticism and clairvoyance to obtain within the realms of the physical universe.   This will be consonant and coherent with ideas of 'hidden' or 'compacted' dimensions, and it sets aside Asiatic and Oriental notions of 'transcendental' entities *manifesting* as men and women.

Ideas of a 'superconscious' will be acceptable to Freudians, as will be the ideas of William James touching upon 'pluralism' and polytheism - under the above provisos. Likewise, the propositions advanced under the aegis of Natural Theology will receive sympathetic consideration.

The ideas of 'mechanistic embodiment', and its close relationship with the structures and function of a warship's computer-based *Intelligent Support System* (aka an ISS), have cogency under the same provisos.   This line of thought brings one close to the Command of a warship and the necessary faculties of *discernment* and *discrimination* of religion.

This is acceptable to the MacKay model.   David Stafford Clark, a Freudian Catholic analyst writes on religion as a (kind of) fall-back position after failure or success of psycho-analysis when the patient finds himself alone in the universe, so to speak.   However, the modern Freudian, in the person of Ethel Spector Person, adopts a more encouraging tone in writing on Love. As does the existentialist Rollo May .

HEALTH – MENTAL AND PHYSICAL

The notion of a SUPERCONSCIOUSNESS is related in at least four ways to thoughts of the 'overall health' of a whole being or organism.   The idea can be found in four different quarters [no pun intended]. First, J.B. Priestley reports on thoughts from a group of medicos, during the Second World War, making use of the term (p. 309)

Second, William James (I seem to remember) made use of the term in his volume, *The Varieties of Religious Experience,* and, likewise, Ludwig von Bertalanffy implies such a notion in one of his volume. William Johnston certainly uses the term in *The Inner Eye Of Love, (p. 187)*, in which he writes (in regard of the word *energy*) 'I am thinking of the Japanese *ki* the Chinese *chi* and the Sanskrit *prana*'.

William Johnston continues: 'all these words point towards a certain cosmic energy or *Life Force* coursing through the whole universe, linking all things together, and coursing also through the whole human body when it is healthy'. The East Asian approach is found pre-eminently in Oriental medicine; and this brings us to the illustrious 'Peckham experiment' in England.

The experiment was conducted by Drs. G. Scott Williamson and Innes H. Pearse between 1926 and 1951, and the 'unswerving preoccupation' of the former is captured, with 'loving and comprehending care', by Dr. Innes Pearse in, *SCIENCE, SYNTHESIS AND SANITY*. Both doctors believed that only a new language could reflect the novel nature of the ideas leading to their success.

I reproduce just two paragraphs of their book (p. 257) which I feel will suffice

Though 'psyche' in its most general sense has to be closely associated with love, the source and origin of which we here attribute to eclectivity in Will, psyche has acquired so many and devious associations that we foresee only further confusion arising from any attempt to make use of the term in this treatise.

Were we, in another sense, expression of man's intuition of being in Memory-Will – then 'soul' might reasonably be equated with the functionary. In that interpretation the artist, poet, mystic, theologian – and the scientist, might well find a future meeting place – i.e. in their location in the dimension Memory-Will.

HIDDEN DIMENSIONS (Time, Space, Mysticism, Religion, Mathematics)

Time

Dimensions of Time have for many decades been the interest of mathematical physicists. They were first 'perceived' by the mathematician and mystic P.D. Ouspensky, whoce ideas were put into practice by a number of illustrious Jungians (see Priestley). Unfortunately, they made the 'Jungian error' of believing Self-Improvement to be an end in itself (except for bringing Meaning into the 'Darkness'). Rudy Rucker appreciates Ouspensky in his book, *The Fourth Dimension...*, (see Rucker).

Space

ESP, related to Time dimensionality, was investigated and reported upon by J.B. Priestly, who also introduced his own personal experience into the discussion. He also cited the mathematical paper presented to the Royal Society by the mathematician and business man, J.G. Bennett, whose paper dwells upon 'manifolds in five-dimensional space'.

Mysticism & Religion

The subject of Mysticism is bifid - natural language dictionaries seldom, if ever, link Mysticism with Religion. Therefore, we have to establish a sub-set of 'Religious' mysticism. I am reluctant to venture into this field – as I allow only natural religion in my systems theoretical approach. But, Hinduism and Jungianism absolutely *demand* that I do so.

This can be restricted, however by considering only phenomena that appear to be *physical*, in which case they will be probably in so-called compacted dimension, i.e. close to the Planck limits of Space and of Time along the *Axis of Scale*. At present, some of the compacted dimensions remain to be determined.

As an example of this we have, in Hindu yoga tradition, the 'spirit' body of the lowest realm of divinity manifesting in the causal and Astral realms as Yin and Yang so as to produce women and men in the material realm. This is so that they can pursue a 'shared karma' or some other form of karma. Power for this (as I understand it) comes from 'Chakras' in other dimensions.

Now, it seems credible that, as the Higgs field is scalar (i.e. non-directional) and permeates all space, it might just be extremely useful in mediating the transmission of power from the causal level to the material level. We could, perhaps, visualize the level as being in the realm of protons and fermions; and it would be interesting to place it along the Axis of Scale. Speculations of this nature are openly bruited abroad by theoretical physicists.

HIERARCHY

There is a loose divide between people who are inclined to think in terms of circularity and those who conceive of think in terms of linearity and hierarchy. This separation may be reflected in differences between East and West, but is seems more likely that it reflects a human propensity in cognition of a lower and more general kind which crosses all such boundaries.

F. David Peat captures the nature of the physical universe well (p. 295):

Nature, therefore, involves a whole series of hierarchies, each one appearing as a tiny adjustment or correction to an underlying level...The universe we live in is a very fine correction, an almost negligible decoration upon the underlying superstring theory.

There may well be many contributing factors at work, such as deontic, normative, sociological, religious, and so on. It is singularly striking that the feminine *type* that appears to be exquisitely and exclusively *carnal* appears to hold no suspicion of regard for hierarchy except for men and women who are within their circle of acceptability.

Jung, one feels, might have considered 'Carmen' rather than 'Eve' in his hierarchy of symbols of womanhood; especially in his portrayal of the nature of the Animus/Anima. Jung could not do any such thing, because he was being forced by his nature, nurture, and particular relationships with women to concoct a completely unreasonable and unrealistic set of Symbols.

David Peat's description is of the hierarchical universe – if not of hierarchical Existence – but it is consonant with the Axis of Scale or Popper's Table of Reductionism. The description encompasses the first set of Realms along that axis, and the relativities are close between this arrangement and that of *Hinduism* (the yogic tradition) and, also, Timothy O'Neill's slant (perspective) on *Jungian theory*.

HIGGS PARTICLE

The higgs particle is a *neutral heavy particle* – not yet found with certainty – which has *very* special properties. There might be one Higgs particle or there might be a family of Higgs particles. There is a 'Higgs field', and 'the quanta of a field are a set of particles'.

Its properties are that it gives (it is thought) different properties to different particles. 'It is as if to some particles the Higgs field is is like a heavy oil through which they move sluggishly and seem to be massive. To other particles the Higgs is like water, and to still others, such as photons and perhaps neutrinos, it is invisible (Lederman, p. 373).

Another way of regarding Higgs is in terms of *symmetry*. The symmetry is exposed at high temperatures, but it is broken at lower temperatures. A metaphor is provided by a magnet which is so because, at low temperatures, its atomic magnets are aligned. It has lost the symmetry of a piece of nonmagnetic iron in which all spatial directions are equivalent.

However, by raising the temperature we can change the magnetic iron into nonmagnetic iron. Lederman remarks that the old, discarded twentieth-century aether has been replaced by a new Higgs field, whose full dimensions we do not yet know.

We *do* know that at least some of the particles representing the Higgs aether must have zero spin, they must be intimately (and mysteriously) connected with mass, and they must manifest themselves at temperatures equivalent to a particular critical energy level (p. 375).

Concerning its structure. One school of thought says it is a fundamental particle. Another school asserts that it is composed of new quark-like objects which might be seen eventually in a laboratory. A third school is intrigued by the possibility of it being in a 'bound state'. In short, the new aether is a 'reference frame for energy'.

HINDUISM   (for Mechanisms and Structures see Motoyama)

The yogic tradition of *Hinduism* asserts that the purpose of all existence is an ongoing evolution that ultimately results in attainment of the Absolute (or unification with God) and that human beings die and are reborn repeatedly until they have reached this goal. It asserts, also, that *inside* the physical universe Yin and Yang operate on and in separate individuals.

The principle that governs this process of reincarnation is the law of cause and effect, or 'karma', as it is generally known (Motoyama, p. 2). For Plato, this is 'metempsychosis; for Jung, it is the result of the 'wrong we have done, thought, or intended' wrought in vengeance on our souls (p.304).

Similar operations and processes are extant In terms of Computer Systems (see PROCESS).

HOLISTIC DUALISM

Whereas Dualism, today, prefers to discriminate between *properties* rather than *substances*, Richard Matterssich adopts an attitude to it which smacks of materialism and academia, without bothering about Science (including, of course, Mathematics. This approach is not only dubious and may also introduce even an element of danger.

An alternative way of regarding common sense is to view it as stemming from Evolutionary Psychology, wherein the evolved brain and its mind (software) and Ego-function, i.e. the evolved 'brain/mind(Ego)', have grown, so to speak, from 'first principles' exhibited even in protozoa. Roger Penrose involves the paramecium [I am rather fond of Chlamydomonas]

These little creatures have their actions decided not only by their circumstances in the world about them but also by their internal state(s) and needs. It can be argued (and it *has* been argued) that such lowly organisms have a *need* for Togetherness as well as needs for survival, nutrition, reproduction, regeneration, encystment, and so on.

Human common sense is multi-facetted. Few people, if any, have complete common sense – it is a matter of strengths and weaknesses in particular areas. The needs for humans are little different – at base – from protozoan needs. And, unfortunately, it is often swayed by sentiment (rather than emotion) or self-interest, etc.

It is closely linked with ability to see clearly *in the correct context.* I have put this in bold lettering because it is so vitally important. If one cannot put thoughts (propositions) into context, one cannot get *the right perspectivel.* If an event or situation is seen from the wrong perspective, then it cannot be *categorized* properly. And, if this is the case, then any organism can be in very great danger.

Ludwig von Bertalanffy writes on such matters, and he even hypothesizes that that the mind/body problem may be shown one day to have so 'difficult' because of erroneous categorization (1973, pp. 252-61). A case in point is Mattessich's argument for 'holistic dualism' whereby he asserts that matter and mind are 'like two faces of one and the same entity' (p. 312).

129

Mattessich is particularly interesting over this. He refers to 'sub-nuclear particles', and to the level of elementary particles as being 'at the bottom of the scale (rather like Popper's declension in *The Self and Its Brain*), but his categorization seems questionable. Mattessich, in fact, appears to suffer (in my opinion) from a touch too much of arrogance and self-belief.

For example, his origins lie in accounting theory and management science (p. xi) , from which (plus further experience) he proceeded to form a Methodology for a dual approach to systems theory which involved 'methods of cognition' and depicting 'means-ends' relationships 'in a holistic setting'.

As a scientist, I find him very short on Science and very long on academic theory. For me, his five 'system principles', and the corresponding 'ontological assumptions', together with the statement that '*the representation of reality makes sense only if all of it, also the realm of value judgments, is taken into account*' (his italics) are the only things of interest.

One feels that Plato's 'common sense' might, today, have said these things without any recourse to computers. But, Mattessich makes no mention of Plato He refers to subjective probability, but only over two pages (pp. 189-190), and he only mentions L.J. Savage and not I.J. Good the creator of a 'landmark in statistical history' (see Savage).

In contradistinction to Mattessich, Karl Popper suggests a Realm of 'sub-sub-atomic particles' might obtain and that new lights might be thrown on the nature of probability. He thinks it worthy of mention that a great biologist [in 1906] reported that 'observation of the behaviour of an amoeba created in him the impression that it was conscious'.

Popper suggests that 'newly emergent entities – both macro and micro – change the *propensities* in their neighbourhood' (p. 30) by introducing new *possibilities* or *probabilities* or *propensities* into that neighbourhood: they create *new fields of propensities*, as when a new star creates a new field of gravitation.

Although Mattessich might seem to cover this in his five systems principles and ontological assertions, there is a wealth of difference between the two perspectives. Mattessich's scheme is closed – it stop at the possibility of a 'leak' (his term) of a field but this is nothing like the reality-changing notion advanced by Popper, which is, in comparison 'wide open'.

HOLOGRAPHY

Roger Penrose reflects, somewhat wryly, that the phenomenon of Holography has become suddenly the 'Holographic Principle'. Opinions differ in mathematical physics about this so-called Principle, but it is critically important in the field of psychotherapy wherein strange and, possibly, abhorrent things are happening. A wide-ranging (but not critical) account is given by Michael Talbot in *The Holographic Universe*.

There are good things and bad things within the matter, but as good account as any, for my purposes, is given by Lee Smolin (p.178) who writes:

The world must be a network of holograms, each of which contains coded within it information about the relationships between the others. In short, the holographic principle is the ultimate realization of the notion that the world is a network of relationships. Those relationships are revealed by this new principle to involve nothing but information.

And, as I type these words, so words are being bandied about relating to information being used and treated in so-called 'superinformation media', 'quantum foam', individual neutrinos being 'far more energetic than those from the sun', and 'u-bits' in complex numbers. The good old Higgs boson seems almost 'old hat', in comparison.

The notion of such a principle was very strong in the middle of the 20th. Century when it was named 'information mechanics', which dealt with things such as 'information interaction', 'information pressure', and so on. Now, as then, claims that the new principle involves nothing but information fall short of their target. They beg numerous questions concerning purpose, utility, hierarchy, level, and, particularly, structure.

We can return to normal, however, by observing that among mathematical physicists there seems to be an increasing number who are dissatisfied with the notion of collapsing wave functions; and this, of course, matches with our mathematical Platonism.

From the perspective of Systems Theoretic 'Perspectivism' and 'Isomorphism' there is significance to be found in Plato's notion of everything being reducible to minute triangles and other geometric figures. Roger Penrose's 'spin networks', etc., and the containment of information offered by the Holographic Principle as it is offered by Smolin readily come to mind.

However, it *is* open to misinterpretation and misuse. This is the case, particularly, in psychological and psychiatric applications. But, it is noteworthy that applications to the boundaries and borders of the physical universe are consistent and coherent with the envisaged separating out of Realms along the Axis of Scale.

'I'

Danah Zohar avers that 'I' am a composite of my relationships [God forbid]. She puts much store in wave-particle duality, and the set of each person's relationships formulates a corresponding set of bosons that acts upon a set of fermions in the way that a ghostly hand strikes a chord on a material piano.

However, there must be, one feels, some *ideal form* shaping the 'hand' that strikes the chords – and that does not seem part of her plan for Pantheism. It is not nearly so neat and simple as is Platonism. With mathematical Platonism everything is fixed, and an 'individual' would be a wave of excitation sweeping through the fixed realm of mathematics and ideal forms.

There would be a need for some mechanism to formulate and to fix the direction of the wave, but it is unlikely to be the untreated whole set of that person's relationships. The sweep of the wave would quite lowly in origin – say the operating system of the earth's living system 'Gaia' or of the solar system. And, conceivably, it would have something to do with the individual's hierarchical set of karmas (see Motoyama).

I – the 'person' or 'personality' writing these words – am, in the words of Ruth Munroe, the 'I' of common parlance. In Freudian terms, I am an Ego-function (but I don't feel fictive). I am well aware of my Id-function – it drives my hormones periodically to fancy 'that girl' (although I don't really want sexual intercourse with her and I may not even know her – see *Sex*)..

If 'that girl' offered me sex I might have a struggle with Self 3, who would remind me that I *love* another. If Self 3 lost the struggle, and I *did* have sex with 'that girl', then I really wouldn't enjoy the sex fully, and I would feel 'soiled' afterwards. Self 3, of course, *has* loved others *but not at this level and not in this way*

It seems to me that Jung was confused about his ego. For example, he considered it in reference to a God with human characteristics that matched his own, he assumed that personality 'surely signifies character' (p. 67). Jung felt the strongest resistance to the comparison of his own ego to that of God (p. 67), but he was a child, and these were his school years.

There are several other noteworthy features mentioned in the previous paragraph. First, and primary, that beyond reasonable doubt Personality resides in the brain/mind(Ego). Second, that Jung had the very human assurance and self-belief that his experiences were unique – they were far from unique, indeed they are commonplace.

Self 2 is more aware of input from Self i than of input from Self 3. This may be that Self 3 is not a product of the brain/mind. There is good evidence that a *Superconscious* zone exists in space-time – in *Hidden Dimensions* – but less evidence that it is transcendental. If so, the Superconscious is ruled out, per se, from levels of divinity (see Motoyama; Johnston).

It is more likely that Self 2 experiences a multiple input from Self 3, from its Animus/Anima, from a transcendental God (along the lines of Natural Theology), from a polytheistic God (William James), or some mizture of them simultaneously.

We have to remember (i) Jung's notion of a tacit belief among scientists in an 'uncomprehended transcendental object that influences and affects us', (ii) that propositions can be assessed, in principle, upon quantitative weights of evidence, and (iii) the importance of experience in such matters. See *Selves*.

IDENTITIES AND SELVES

Composite

Individual

INDIVIDUATION

Had Jung fully embraced ideas from the East he would not have misconceived Individuation. This process is absolutely normal and natural within the physical universe because it relates to some ommand element gaining mastery of the lower-grade vessel which serves it. The Commander of a warship, for example, spends years gaining that knowledge and experience – both practical and theoretical – which entitles him to full operational Command.

Therefore, in the physical universe (when Yin and Yang are operating separately and independently) that subsystem which has Command responsibility within a man or a woman 'Individuates' by gaining sufficient operational maturity and expertise to pursue its major goal or karma. Once this has been done the so-called 'spiritual' entity once more – if all karmas have been satisfied – contains the Yin and Yang principles within its bounds.

Progress along those lines is indicated by William James (and by Donald MacKay) in relation to mystical indwelling, union, and merger; but 'ordinary' people often get piecemeal experiences of 'partial' states.

INDWELLING AND MERGER

Amid a myriad of verbiage over *Love* and *Mysticism*, one finds occasionally the concept of Male and Female – free, material 'poles' of one higher, Spiritual, entity co-operating together in order to supply it with their *shared* experiences of the same phenomena. The construct can be focussed down, so to speak, to Hinduism in its yogic form. See Motoyama; Johnston.

Such an arrangement, per se, is not uncommon in systems theory but an important point to be made here is, that it relates to *Clairvoyance* and *ESP*, and the difference between them. This pertains to the difference between *Merger* and *indwelling* (which involves, also, the difference between Buddhism and Christianity). See William Johnston.

The indwelling phenomenon is not telepathy so much as it is instantaneous shared experience from different perspectives, so as to give 'fullness'. It squares with MacKay's ideology in Comprhensive Realism, and with Hinduism and Jung's notions of the Animus/Anima (but only as they are represented by Timothy O'Neill). It is *Experiential*.

The *reality* of such an occurrence can be established beyond all reasonable doubt if the event contains, within itself and common to both entities, something which is unequivocally most highly unlikely and far beyond any kind of synchronicity generated from, say, some relational and/or associative database.

Not surprisingly, such occasions are rare; and this has been pointed out by Motoyama and by Jung in their different ways. Additionally, Motoyama has pointed out that, in regard of computers, one small event (say, a change in the sign of one 'bit') can have a most drastic effect. It is noted, re Complexity theory, as the Butterfly effect.

It follows, in essence, that one small phenomenon can possess an enormous 'weight of evidence' provided it is perceived or specificated within the appropriate context and related to the apposite theme.

INEXPLICABLE FEATURES

The paradigm that I offer has very mechanistic features, such as mathematical Platonism and the mechanistic embodiment of mathematical formulae, but this is not exhaustive. Nevertheless, many of the biological processes of which we are aware can be traced 'down' to formal logico-mathematics. Ludwig von Bertalanffy gives many examples.

It is possible to trace certain features of Nature 'upwards' – in the sense that 'downwards' categorization sometimes produces a particular instance of something, within a category, that is simply inexplicable: it just cannot be reconciled with any characteristics of the category and we are forced to reconsider the categorization process that led to the discovery.

This is a vital part of human cogitation, and occasionally we find that the inexplicable phenomenon leads to fresh conjectures – and their acceptance – in a totally different direction and from an unforeseen perspective. This kind of sea-change does not come easily to human thinking. Many of us, if not most, like to follow up remorselessly a 'good idea'.

It is necessary, therefore, to distinguish between those modes of perception and judgment which apply to all living things, i.e. organisms, and those which are exclusively or predominantly human characteristics. And, in this respect, it seems likely that I.J. Good's version of subjective probability was under-rated by Savage. Good contributed not only to Statistics, but also to the Judgment and Perception of Everyman and Everywoman.

By his concept of 'degrees of belief', Good provided a basis for the logico-mathematical nature of all living things, and enables us to conceive of this fundamental quality of life being swamped by, and lost in, the organa of thought posited in succession by Aristotle, Bacon, and Ouspensky in terms of logic that is deductive, Inferential, and Intuitive.

However, this sequence can be extended further by interpreting the term, logic, as 'a means of gaining knowledge'. Thereafter, several forms of 'mystical knowledge become acceptable because we are working with degrees of belief. These forms range from propinquity (togetherness as two individuals), through union (as a pair, i.e. a relation between 'poles'), up to what is called 'mystical indwelling'. And, they then (now) include such things as telepathy, precognition, and 'simultaneous apperception of the same phenomenon'.

For convenience, the latter case may be called 'clairvoyance', and it can be scrutinized and evaluated in terms of plausibility and degrees of belief – by all and sundry, not just applied statisticians.   In other words, we can revive and restore the 'natural common sense' that has become subjugated but not extinguished.

In general, we can counter superstitious nonsense, which extends into and affects all walks of life, by sets of belief that are formally part of Nature.   To give a specific example, we can counter the deleterious taradiddle of whole societies obsessed with 'ghosts and ghoulies' by common sense in terms of plausible existing 'availabilities'.

Any conventional understanding of a 'ghost', for instance, can be understood completely in terms of the 'chakras' and 'nadis' of Hindism which are held to possess, in the form of the human body, an 'astral body' which obtains in the 'hidden dimensions' of the 'astral plane'.   All such considerations of which come into the realm of particle physics and are supported by phenomenal facts of the yoga tradition (see Motoyame; Johnston).

This illustrates how phenomena which are 'inexplicable in one scenario can become explicable in another, and it emphasizes the critical importance of categorization – as is promoted in von Bertalanffie's logico-mathematical 'General System Theory'.   And, in reference to that domain, there are several noteworthy points – all of which are interlinked features of it-

The first of these is that Ervin Laszlo, with his unified field theory, is seen by certain people in systems theory as as the natural successor to Ludwig von Bertalanffy (see Mattessich).   The second point is that this is joined by the constructs of Hinduism and of particle physics to Jungian theory.   The third point is that these notions are all encompassed and explained by the various concepts of Dimensionality which can all be deemed 'hidden dimensions'.

For example, we can list 'compacted dimensions', posted by physicists to make quantum mechanics 'neat and tidy'.   Also to be listed, there is the concept of the *time* dimensions seen as necessary by Ouspensky to accommodate intuitive logic or *tertium organum* (and by others for various reasons).

Particularly valuable is the concept of *Scale* as a dimension posted by mathematician Rudy Rucker, which has enabled the constructs of many others to be sited along an *Axis of Scale*.   This is the construct which we perceive now to embrace the whole of Existence – so far as it can be conceived – from the material realm to the structured orders of Infinity and the Transfinite as they were discovered (just over a century ago) by Georg Cantor.

It is just conceivable that we may eventually come to see Emotion as another dimension.   This has been floated (ephemerally) by a varied number of people, but the idea of emotional information was given us by von Bertalanffy.   A similar notion was taken up by Clynes, under the term *Sentics*.

Yet again, Solomon shows us how the Passions may be broken down into characteristic sets of descriptors, and, of course, computers are just the thing for all such perspectives on the mechanization of mind-like processes.   Livesey, furthermore, ties emotion into heuristic learning through the process of Evolution.

INNER SELF

A phrase used by Popper and Eccles approximating to a Soul or Command Element.

ISOMORPHISM

Systems Theory, in the persons of Ludwig von Bertalanffy and Richard Mattessich, makes much over *isomorphism*, but a few simple sketches with pen and paper show that the idea should be treated with some care – especially when extension into other dimensions is concerned (it really is a matter of common sense related to topology).

Specifically, isomorphism is defined as 'two systems in widely differing fields having the same flow-diagrams'. Ludwig von Bertalanffy (1973, pp. 80-86) writes of 'isomorphism of laws' in science. He suggests that there are three pre-requisites for isomorphisms in different fields and sciences, and remarks that the isomorphisms of laws rests upon both our cognition and the nature of reality.

The subject of isomorphism is relevant to the notions of Archetypes and to the concepts of Ideal Forms. As did Jung with archetypes, so von Bertalanffy asserts that 'the number of simple mathematical expressions which will be preferably applied to describe natural phenomena is limited', hence, he argues, laws identical in structure will appear in intrinsically different fields.

The same argument is made about statements made in ordinary language, but one must have some doubts about its rigour in view of the 'collapsing wave-function' construct in physics and concept from subjective probability of natural language propositions having numerical 'degrees of belief' (provided they arise from a consistent and coherent 'body of beliefs'.

Nevertheless, Ludwig von Bertalanffy's description of three different levels in the description of phenomena is useful. The trio indicates limitations imposed by the *assumption* of principles underlying isomorphism in different realms. In ascending order of power they are: *analogies*, *homologies*, and the third level of *Explanation*. And, clearly, this third level fits very neatly with subjective probability's notions of the numerical weighting of propositions.

Richard Mattessich says much the same thing (p. 322). His language is more 'high falooting' (i.e. esoteric and convoluted) but there is no clear distinction between them – other than that. Indeed, in essence he endorses von Bertalanffy's *Perspectivism* by saying 'the *difference between a fact and a norm hinges on the point of view* from which a system is looked at' (his italics).

A down to earth 'practical and pertinent' example, which tallies (in parts) with experience, is given by evolutionary psychology. From the lowliest (protozoa) to the highest (humans), organisms appear to have some faculty for grouping together, and we can consider the *theme* of relationship, which some claim to be a universal and sole existent.

If our starting point is taken as the lowest conjectural proposition, i.e. Whitehead's concept of 'Togetherness' giving a 'subjective aim for 'Concrescence', then we can consider 'variations' on this theme in regard of their being representable by just one diagram.

So, we find Plato's 'affinitive search' – two parts of one soul seeking each other – for re-union with God; the Yin and the Yang as sub-principles of a spiritual Life Force driving a 'Spirit-Body'; Jung's Life Force driving a spirit body subdivided into the Logos and Eros; MacKay's embodied formulae merging and melding; Johnston's mystical merging and indwelling, and countless mythical and literary representations (see the Appendix).

All of which points up Jung's quaint notion of 'internal completion'. It is clear that this idea is not so much 'quaint' as it was *enforced* by the constraints imposed upon him by (his choice of) life style and his childhood experiences – reinforced by his personality weaknesses.

The concept of isomorphism, supported by quantitative appraisal from subjective probability and information theory, does lend credence to the concept embraced by both von Bertalanffy and by Mattessich. But, as said elsewhere in this monograph, the construct needs to be approached with care.

JUNGIAN THEORY (My emphases throughout)

Jung claimed that every judgment made by an individual is conditioned by his personality type and that every point of view is necessarily relative (1964, p. 198). He revealed that his life had been 'permeated and held together' by one idea and one goal, namely, 'to penetrate into the secret of the personality'. Furthermore, he explained: 'Everything can be explained from this central point, and all my works relate to this one theme' (p. 197).

As one who is not without knowledge in the field of 'The Influence of Personality upon Information-Processing Systems', I assert that Jung was wrong. He was wrong not over the attributes and functions, but over the purposes and location of Personality. And this largely reduces the quality and cogency of the whole Jungian opus.

Because every attribute and function (major and minor) of Personality, as it is seen by Jung, is equally typical of a real-time military computer system, I refer to the mind and its identity, the Ego, as being *encephalized*. That term was not coined by me and, for convenience, I use the term when referring to the *brain/mind(Ego)* in reference to a neurophysiological *mental system*.

It follows that the encephalization process produces a large number of 'models', and these are open to use as analogues, test-beds, bases for experimentation, or (as I have done) linguistic analysis by computer. Details of an experiment yielding significant results are given in the Appendix.

KARMA AND REBIRTH

Plato

Hindu Yogic

Karma can apply to Relationships as in 'shared karmas'

LIFE FORCE

Jung

Hinduism

LIKELIHOOD

See 'MATHEMATICS and STATISTICS' in the Bibliography

(For a definition of the term and a worked example see 'Brownlee')

LOVE AND SEX

Love is clearly a 'force' within the physical universe for the eminent C.S.Sherrington, neuro-physiologist. He associates Love with Nature and Evolution. We know this because, among other things, he states, boldly and categorically, that *Nature's Aim* is 'Altruism as Passion' and that man 'must love wherever Love can be felt'.

He says little about Sex, but asserts – over a whole chapter – that brain collaborates with psyche. There are great similarities between his dualistic hypothesis and the *'strong dualistic hypothesis'* advanced by Popper and Eccles. They inform us that Sherrington did not at first believe that psyche survived death, but later changed his mind.

Whereas they hold a naïve view of the User of a computer being the programmer, Sherrington holds exactly the right concept of the User (i.e. the psyche) to match impeccably with the real-time computer system serving the captain of a vessel of war. His concept of man's environment (a 'battlefield' far and wide) is absolutely appropriate, and his notion that the brain's operations converge towards a kind of 'decision-making point' is identical with the warship's computer system.

All of this identifies the organism and the warship with a Mission (or Missions) orientated towards the Other and as part of Nature (Altruism as Passion). This figures – because the chain of Command requires only the ability to give the 'Command fiat' down a hierarchy of authority.

We see that Sherrington did not see the possibility of Altruism as Passion arising from the material organic body by way of Evolution. His ideas were put forward under the aegis of Natural Theology – so there is no discrepancy there, provided we accept the psyche as being non-transcendental.

In fact, he *does* identify the psyche with a *mental system* (p. 260) geared to 'all that counts in life (p. 266), namely desire, zest, truth, love, knowledge, and values'. The values, we note, take us from 'hell's depth to heaven's utmost height'. But, as he points out, the psyche is not part of experience'.

How then, we might ask, can the psyche not be part of experience? Simple! The psyche has access to Experience. Therefore, we can perhaps conjecture that the Platonic concept of the psyche as the pilot of a ship holds good. Popper and Eccles think so.

With two of the greatest neuro-physiologists who ever lived arguing so broadly in line with each other – backed up so strongly by computer models – who can say Nay? Ernest Kent can do so. However, his monistic argument is based, surprisingly, upon a misconception of computer systems. His case is founded upon the 'Supervisor' part of the software system being able to conduct looking ahead activities that are part of a much more advanced system.

As this software is part of the triune brain which evolves into exactly those Supervisor – Operating System duties, Kent's only strength lies in supporting the two dualistic hypotheses from a different perspective.

In short, it seems likely that both Sex and Love are properties of the physical universe in the same way that Language is a property. That is to say, they are part and parcel of physical existence. In a way, we can go no further than that in definition, because we cannot even – at the lowest level – give adequate definitions of Living or Non-Living (see, for example, Taxonomy).

This may well involve 'Hidden Dimensions' and be dependent, also, on the level at which the relevant functions operate in the hierarchy of, say, emotional complexity. With Sex we have a drive for reproduction geared to periodicity of hormone production. With Love, there are manifestations of Togetherness rising to the point of self-sacrifice.

Plato seems able to describe the state of loving, but it may be that he had his tongue in his cheek (see Joan Wynn Reeves). All in all, descriptions of Love are best left to the poets; and, for that reason, they are contained in the Appendix. An alternative source is William Johnston's work on Mysticism.

Recourse to the natural quaternion gives an illustration of the sociological differences between Love and Sex. Sexual activities vary in acceptability between cultures and over different periods of time, whereas Love is broadband (except in the unfortunate world of Screwtape).

MANIFESTATION and IMPLEMENTATION

There is very little difference, in essence, between the Hindu notion of a person as a *manifestation* in the material Realm engineered by the Yin or the Yang principle and the placement of the contents of a program into the CPU or 'working space' of a computer (as distinct from 'memory', 'services, etc.). The material body has to be 'driven' and the program has to be 'activated'.

The activated program is a process stretching – in terms of Causality – from the 'Client', for whom the 'Programmer' worked, to the dismantling of each word in the program and the setting into hardware-motion of each designated part of each word. That process incorporates all four of Aristotle's forms of Causality.

The process also embraces three different kinds of Time, and it is not difficult to imagine these as being orthogonal to each other – just as Ouspensky envisaged dimensional Time. This scheme has been put into mathematical form by P.D. Bennett (and his colleagues), but it has been tied into experience by J.B. Priestley.

The individual 'Times' of the process can be called, re Computer systems, 'User Time', 'Machine Time', and 'Conversion Time' (as the *potential* in the program's instruction sequence is changed into *real* mechanical activity. A number of 'correction factors' are appropriate to sharpen up this particular perspective, such as scale, and they can then be fitted imaginatively into Bennett's terminology of 'PassingTime', 'Eternity', and 'Hyparxis'. (see Priestley).

Such ideas sit easily, also, with Alister Hardy's concept of a driver in charge of a railway engine. Or, Roger Delgado's remote control over a bull. It is worthy of note that the notion of time-dimensions has occupied the minds of theoretical physicists for many decades, and that interest is being heightened today by the phenomenon of non-locality.

MEANING

The encephalization of Personality effectively transposes the Mind(Ego) from the non-material Jungian *psyche* to the material living world and its evolutionary stream. The psyche remains, but it now functions as the Command element of a 'vessel', i.e. the body of a living organism (there are likely to be non-material parts of the organism which may or may not include the Command element).

This brings Jungian theory appreciably closer to Natural Theology, in which case we can view the Command element as Sherrington's 'ultimate pontifical nerve-cell' and expect Jung's 'hints from the unconscious' and 'sudden decisive impulses' to be physical and mystical (in hidden dimensions) rather than transcendental. It also makes us wonder about the purpose underlying Life.

Jung's concept of that purpose being 'to bring light into the darkness of mere being' has all sorts of theological implications, but it is plausible. However, a shorter-term, more immediate, purpose, would be to make ethical decisions while steering the vessel through waters muddied by interactions between the sex drive hidden in the 'natural quaternion' and 'the social Leviathan', so as to achieve the highest goal of all. The notions of William James and of William Johnston then assume considerably more status.

The concepts of Ethel Spector Person and of Rollo May also become prominent through the former's concept of 'Love as an agent of change' and the latter's belief that sexual polarity is an 'ontological necessity'. These ideas, together with other beliefs that human bodies are 'action systems', or 'embodied formulae', or 'we are all "stories", etc., begin to show coherence.

MISSION AND COMMAND

For Plato, a person's 'mission' was to achieve re-union between his/her 'part-soul' (psyche) with its missing 'part'; and, in the material 'world', this process is a very mechanistic and *cybernetic* business involving cyclicity, periodicity, control, feedback, and the all-important *goal* of re-union.

There was, for Plato, an element of choice in this: a man could either follow the path of 'the Good' or he could opt not to do so. If he chose continually the 'not-Good' path, then metempsychosis would eventually reduce him to some appropriate animal.

The mechanics of this are similar to the way processes are treated in a warship. If a process continually fails to perform as has been specified in their ideal form or *process image*, then either the User or the Chief Design Engineer can eliminate it or alter its powers in some way. Apart from the effects of those two, the process image is inviolate (this is why it has to be copied into the working space).

The parallel can be extended to some extent by designating the warship's overall 'Mission' as the Good (it *is* for the protection and nurturing of Others), and by seeing the succession of minor tasks as an 'itinerary' or some kind of 'working up' process – self-protection is necessary to achieve the Good.

This is a self-regulating and self-referential process, because the individual, for Plato, carries with him/her the recollection of the Other (part-soul) and, thus, it can foresee its Mission-fulfilment in *the Anticipated Whole Other*. Unfortunately, this utterly plausible conjecture is rejected by Jungians in favour of a _real_ picture of a _fictive_ woman built up by the accumulation of a myriad of impressions of women, encountered over aeons of time, _to be discarded_ after use.

The encephalization of the Mind(Ego) makes an enormous difference to Jung's ideology. It rids the mind-set of Ruth Munroe's 'mystical balderdash' (but not quite the same constructs as she perceived), and it makes what is left not only palatable but pertinent to daily life *and* to scientific and philosophical discourse.

For example, our feelings of subordinacy, or of being 'characters in stories', and so on, seem genuine and authentic in terms of Ego-awareness generated by a material brain/mind(Ego) that is an evolved 'Intelligent Support System'. In MacKay's terms, the brain/mind(Ego) is the *Agent* and the superordinate system, operating through the Zoharian interface, is the *Determinator*. Both constructs lie within an embodied mathematical formula, and both are open to external pushes and pulls.

[see also Moral Responsibility]

MORAL RESPONSIBILITY

All of Jung's confusion and inconsistency (and obfuscation) comes to a head, one might say, in his Chapter (in MDR) on Late Thoughts – some twenty-four pages. He asserts, correctly, that to have an answer to evil we must 'know relentlessly' – without self-deception or self-delusion – how much good we can do and the crimes of which we are capable.

Jung goes on to posit a fundamental stratum or core of human nature wherein dwell the instincts. Here, says Jung, are pre-existent dynamic factors which ultimately *govern* [my italics] our ethical conscious decisions (p. 305). It gets worse – nothing, says he, can spare us the torment of ethical decisions from which, in the future, the creative determinant visits upon our souls the wrongs that we have 'done, thought, or intended' (p. 304).

Abrogating Love to God (as cosmogonic love), introduces the notions of 'duty' and 'conflict of duties'. He does this having swept away 'self-evident' categories of Good and Evil when, on the previous page (p. 303), he does a pretty good job of defining evil as 'determinant reality'. Referring to a *principle of evil*, he lists naked injustice, tyranny, lies, slavery, and coercion of conscience. Written more than fifty years ago, his words are strikingly reflective of the world of today.

This is not all. His numerous biographers refer amply to his succession of *'femmes inspiratrices'*, and his *persuasion* of his wife to join with his mistress and himself in a *ménage a trois.* If ever a person needed to practice what he preaches it is Jung. Nevertheless, the 'good stuff' is wonderful and admirable.

This bewildering array of inconsistencies is made even more obscure by the fact that the words used by him in reference to moral responsibility and duty fit almost perfectly into a description of Command, as in the Command of a warship or, better, the Pilot of a ship (in the way used by the Classical Greeks to describe a leader into dark and dangerous places, i.e. the psyche). But such a meaning cannot be ascribed to the level of the instincts.

Furthermore, the goal of psychic development as postulated by Jung, is not (as might be expected) Altruism but *the Self.* Sherrington's notion of Nature's Aim being Altruism as Passion is nothing to do with instinct – it is everything to do with the evolution of an 'ultimate *pontifical* nerve cell' [my italics]. There still remains, however, after the *encephalization of the mind(Ego)* a remnant of Jung's original idea of a spiritual Command element that issues the Command fiat.

Nevertheless, with encephalization of the Mind(Ego), Jungian theory becomes vastly improved and extremely useful and comprehensible. However, although sharply observed, his approach to ethical decisions and moral responsibility is shown to be patchy and incomplete.

He is absolutely correct in pointing out that, in daily life, we are faced with incessant encounters with moral decisions and with crises of conscience. He is probably correct in assuring us that any SINS we have *INTENDED* (not 'thought, said, or done) will be visited upon us by the Creative Determinant (i.e. operating system of the local universe).

Furthermore, and for Jung this must have been difficult, he correctly pointed out that we must examine ourselves most rigorously to discover what 'sins' we are capable of (etc.)   Here, there is much room for self-deception – as he displayed when he disagreed with Freud's interpretation of Jung's dream (and Jung 'knew' that he could not have dreamed in that vein).

Even so, Jung appears to have discerned correctly one essential element of the Command function – that is to take full responsibility (under the terms and conditions stated above) for his actions.   But now, under an encephalized Mind(Ego), this responsibility lies with the Ego or SuperEgo and not with any non-material system.

In short, the Ego equates with Ruth Munroe's 'I' of common parlance, with the evolved 'brain/mind(Ego), and with Sherrington's 'ultimate pontifical cell'. And, here, we come to an extremely difficult and important philosophical point about Free Will, which re-introduces MacKay's concept of a *Determinator*.   Also introduced are the nature of sin, purpose and priority, and an Intelligent Support system – as an *Agent* subject to a *Determinator*.

Jung's assertion that accurate and deep self-knowledge is necessary in facing moral dilemmas is, of course, correct - but it is *incomplete*.   And this is an interesting feature, because in view of his notions of superordinacy and psychagogues, daemons, et al., one might have expected a professed empiricist to calibrate, so to speak, his individual histories of advice against the results obtained from taking or rejecting this advice.

This surprise is increased when he remarks that he learned to accept immediately the thoughts, premonitions, forebodings, etc., that come to most people in daily life. Much of this, we know, results from the intake of food and drink.   This quite frequently produces mental antagonisms and/or agonizing over trivia.

However, there are occasions wherein normative and deontic issues <u>are </u>at stake. An example is when a man or women is badly jilted and resolves to 'go to the devil' – and then finds that he/she cannot take the necessary first step in that direction. Alternatively, a man and woman may find themselves in a position that requires them to pursue an undesirable and difficult course of action as a point of honour.   Even today these situations *do* occur; and they are the meat and drink of literary fiction and of poetry (see the Appendix).

Thus, it seems from such considerations that we must continuously be scrupulously attentive to our actions, and the intentions behind them, - past present and future.   Not in fear but from sheer common sense.   The social Leviathan is always present 'grooming' us for some purpose of its own, and all the so-called 'social media' contain evidence of this, if we look closely enough.   The 'buzz-word' used to be 'Hidden Agenda' but 'Political Correctness' may seem its rival.

MOVING FINGER

Omar Khayyam spoke to his Beloved about the Moving Finger that writes and having writ moves on.   He had, said he, consulted with doctors and with saints and had received no useful advice.   So, he implored the Beloved, let us live for the moment.   Poor Omar – he had read the wrong books and consulted the wrong people.

The books that he should have read had been written by Plato and his pupil, Aristotle; and, had he lived some eight hundred years later, their words would have been backed by systems science, systems technology, and systems philosophy (von Bertalanffy) *and* by contemporary philosopher and scientists, such as Ethel Spector Person and Rollo May.

I pick out those two, in particular, because they argue the power of Love, and I could have mentioned, also, William Johnston. Ethel Person describes Love as an 'agent of change'. Rollo May points out, first, that maleness and femaleness are an 'ontological necessity' and, second, that Love contains an inbuilt 'imperative to act'.

William Johnston describes aspects of relationship concerning mystical union, merger, and indwelling wherein lurks clairvoyance (as distinct from ESP) and shared knowledge and experience. On this, I have some personal experience – enough, for example, to comment upon Jung's visions and personifications, and also to make some useful comment about those things, in general.

Additionally, Omar would be knowledgeable about *programs* and about the *programmers* who write programs for their *clients* – who might also be considered as *'Users'*. He would know that programs can be implemented (used) any number of times and remain unchanged. Alternatively, some programs can be self-referential and change themselves.

Furthermore, Omar would know that (according to current opinion) programs would not be for individuals but for relationships. In this case, it is quite possible that a program could be replayed any number of time to furnish different *perspectives* on any particular relationship. Also, that this could be done in terms of mathematics.

Thus, he and his Beloved could, for example, participate in a shared karma (see Motoyama) or separately to guide each other as twinned poles of one higher entity. In this, I am thinking not only about the Hindu yogic tradition, but also about certain aspects of particle physics and mathematical Platonism. Not to mention, Jungian theory (i.e. the amended theory).

Aristotle's notions of Causality and of system complexity are particularly suited to Computer Systems. All four forms of Causality are present in programs, but in mathematical Platonism a different perspective has to be taken. In this the notion of 'potential' is somewhat different.

MYSTICAL KNOWLEDGE (AND ESP)

I am quite willing to use the term ESP loosely within the concept of Mystical knowledge, because we gain such knowledge from it coming to us through our material sensory apparatus and/or our imagination. In referring to visions, personifications, I make use of William Johnston and Lawrence le Shan.

Dr. Le Shan has been head of a Department of Psychology, and whereas he gathers his 'evidence' on ESP from the observations made by experts across different disciplines in order to seek out phenomenological common facts, I reverse the procedure and take the common facts as the starting place. I do this because, in the field of mystical knowledge and ESP, I can speak from experience *and* from the viewpoint of *statistical likelihood*.

William Johnston, citing William James, lists four characteristics of mystical knowledge given by William James, namely *ineffability, noetic quality, transiency,* and *passivity*. He quotes James on the last of these, passivity: 'the mystic feels as if his own will is in obeyance , and indeed sometimes as if he were grasped and held by a superior power' (James, p. 372).

I am not sure whether or not I am a mystic, but I have had experiences completely in line with ineffability, noesis, transience, and passivity. However, I have some misgivings about passivity. From my own experience (seemingly as an Agent) passivity is more psychological than mystical. Jung seems to have viewed it as, perhaps, Acceptance. In psychological terms (Freudian) I have experienced almost tangible 'grinding' in which the ego goes against the superego *or* vice-versa.

In Jungian terms the experience is as if it were one going against a psychagogue or against one's animus/anima. On this matter of passivity I would plump for Freud — especially in a revamped setting of an encephalized mind(Ego). I cover most of such personal experiences in the Appendix.

MYSTICAL LANGUAGE (AND COMMUNICATION)

William Johnston uses natural language words to describe and explain Mystical Knowledge, but his words are interwoven with religious quotations and references. Lawrence Le Shan uses the natural language opinions of others who are more qualified in Science and Technology; but they do not contradict one another.

Johnston's words on mystical reports, such as Void, Veil, Nothingness, Love, Action, Union, Discernment, etc., are all commonplace and they are all context dependent. I have shown experimentally that words, used as signs (Peircean indexes) and weighted according to context, can lead to experimental subjects simulating (with apparently significant success) situation appraisal at the reptilian level.

But those words, used commonly every day, are also meaningful to me from a mystical perspective [I am not claiming to *be* a mystic] because they relate to my experience. In particular, 'Void' and 'veil' bring to mind particular features of experiences in ESP and/or mysticism that I may, or may not, have interpreted wrongly.

However, these natural language words are not the only medium of communication, and I have in mind Poetry and Music. I have permission from the Folio Society and the Institute of Mathematics to quote freely from their publication on these matters, and this I do on poetry, gratefully, in the Appendix. I can only refer to the field of Music, and *this* I do here by citing Dr. Manfred Clynes and his volume on *Sentics*. I admire greatly *Language and Context* by Elizabeth Bates, especially her introductory pages.

The nature of, and the categorization of, Information is a matter for Systems Theory, Information Theory, Linguistics, Praxeology, and so on; but my coverage of the exchange of information between Ego-consciousness and a hypothesized psychagogue or Anima is open to analysis, which I give in the main text of Part Two. .

MYSTICAL INDWELLING, UNION, MERGER

MYTHS AND LEGENDS

MYTHS AND IRRATIONALITY

Jung bewailed the slumbering and decaying of the myth of Christianity and, thus, aroused hopes of clear thinking in one part of our society while at the same time generating fury and revilement in another. Then, puzzlingly, he asserts that 'the only ray of light is Pope Pious X11 and his dogma' (p. 306), whereby he begs several questions.

Jung's identification of Christian myth as Christian dogma actually raised many questions – both 'laterally and hierarchically. They are not *imponderables*, but they are *insoluble* without qualification. And, one feels that this is but one of the numerous aspects of the human condition. Jung averred that Mankind is raised from the animal world by powers of reflection (p. 312), but there is more to it than that.

For example, Jung referred to Man's use of a 'disciplined imagination' (p. 287), and and Whitehead might have referred to a general 'principle of abstraction'. And, going down to that level of 'basics', the most fundamental question of all is probably, 'Why is there something rather than nothing?'. This relates directly to the myth/dogma identity question.

One answer to the question of Existence is through Man's discovery of mathematics – he discovered or invented 'the empty set'. Nothing (zero) cannot be represented in the chain of natural numbers without the creation of something, i.e. the empty set.

The implications of this are that descriptions of any existing entities cannot be complete or perfect – they are approximate and have to be qualified. They (the descriptions) rest in Man's powers of invention, discovery, insight, intuition, etc., and clearly they relate to the Environment of both the entity and the entity giving the description.

In short, Incompleteness reigns; and Kurt Godel argued this in two 'incompleteness theorems' which use 'purely mathematical reasoning to prove certain facts about the objective world (Rucker, 1982, p. 164). Godel showed that no finitely describable theory can codify all mathematical truth, which is immediately obvious to any machine code programmer using a digital computer and familiar with Cantor's diagonal proof of the Transfinite.

Thus, we come back to the notions of papal dogma as myth, and of the purported myth of Christianity. Again, we find an assertion from Jung which sounds rather odd. He asserts that there is 'a greater territory of the self which lies beyond the section of Christian morality', and that one's soul (his mother's) can be taken into that 'wholeness of nature and spirit in which conflicts and contradictions are resolved' (p. 290).

Allowing for such things as translation difficulties, individualism in the use of words and idiosyncrasies, irrationality (which we all have), 'hang-ups' (which we all have) and so on, this makes almost perfect sense if we relate it to Tom Bombadil and Goldberry (in the terms used by Timothy O'Neill), and to the Hindu yogic tradition (as described by Motoyama).

In this context, Tom Bombadil and Goldberry are mythical characters representing manifestations of a man and a woman in the material world. They are manifested by the principles of Yang and Yin, respectively, with energies originating in a 'spirit body' operating through a 'soul body', Hiroshi Motoyama describes the process, and Walter Mons cites the equivalence to Christian concepts.

In many ways, those two characters are represented in other myths as variations of the category of myth, say, of '*Reunion After Travails*'. Many such versions obtain, such as Odysseus and Penelope, Lancelot and Guinivere, and (subject to debate and to interpretation) Leo Vincey and Ayesha (Compare the original text, in essence, with many 'renditions' of it)

The latter pair, in particular, bring out the fact that they *are* mythical characters and are, therefore, subject to use by anybody for any purpose. Much the same applies to the other pairs, and any *truth* to be found in them is most likely to be that human cognition and ratiocination operate along certain lines.

Under the Jungian aegis – as it is corrected by O'Neiil – Goldberry and Tom Bombadil may be taken loosely as each being individuated and both working together – at the Sapientic level – to work out their joint karma and, thus, to then enable the spirit body to proceed to the levels of divinity.

This is what Jung could not, or would not, include in his ideology, and it becomes crystal clear when the corrected Jungian notions are united with the Sino-Asiatic model (as above) and the resultant is joined further with the Jungian *Personality* embodied in the material level (as was shown in Pt. Two).

Jung took *Meaning*, and the spread of Meaning, as lying behind Man's Purpose; but that idea is not convincing for a number of reasons. A much better one is *Experience* – this has a very broad compass, but it cannot always be defined in terms of Rationality, Irrationality, or any particular life form. The Victorians referred to *the Occult*, and there seems to be no good reason for not using it as a generic term today.

In this region, we venture into the philosophical foundations of competing theories and look for commonality. The exercise is epitheoretical and it involves an 'ideological web', of which this entry is part. We are encouraged in undertaking this task by the findings, and the measures, of subjective probability.

With *Experience*, we are taking first steps towards a so-called 'Semantic web', but the notion of an ideological web is charged with spine-tingling possibilities for putting our *Experience* to good use. Especially, with regard to the ever-increasing speed of computer design and development, together with appropriate essays into Experimental Psychology.

The late Joseph Campbell suggested that a psychological analysis of myths might provide us with a better understanding of their essential qualities, so as to see how they continue to reflect human needs and can assuage anxieties. And this, one feels, can help us to understand Jung's relating of myth to dogma.

NATURAL QUATERNION

The 'natural quaternion' is the quartet of relationships occurring in Nature, wherein three are relational within Biology's living stream (Parent, Offspring, Sibling) and the fourth is 'Other'.

NATURE'S AIM

Sherrington sees this as being 'Altruism as Passion' making us 'Love wherever Love can be felt'.

NETWORKS AND NODES

Current claims that the 'world' is nothing but Information', as I have said elsewhere, are far too shallow and sweeping. And, I will say this immediately because all networks have *nodes*, and Danah Zohar's assertion that 'we are our relationships' is better phrased as 'we are hubs in a myriad of relationships of varying orders and degrees'.

It, too, makes a nonsense of Jung's assertion that we must eschew emotional ties, because the 'world' is nothing but relational *bonds* set out by the natural quaternion and fed upon by the social Leviathan. *Au contraire*, we must seek, devotedly and constantly, to understand our relationships, and to *control* them in the light of our appraisal of them.

This does not mean that we should proselytize. This I deplore and I reject all organized religions because proselytization is their aim; and I *do* have some sympathy with Jung's attitude on this. One has only to examine, for example, a spider's web (with its accretions at the nodes after rainfall) to envisage my meaning.

One could almost call this communications network a 'web' of understanding' in this particular context (after the 'Cloud of Unknowing'), and this is implicit in the 'MacKay model' of Comprehensive Reality. The model, which I endorse and augment, is centred upon the real-time computer system which serves the individual and provides intercommunication between groups of vessels.

In this, I refer to the 'Command, Control, and Communication' centres that operate in support of Task Forces and Fleets and Flotillas by the use of data-links. It seems to me that the idea runs quite close to Jung's concept of the Personal Unconscious, the Racial

Unconscious, and the Collective Unconscious. This comparison has been put to Jungians (not by me) and it has met with some approval. It is one more aspect of the Warship Analogy.

In addition to the social and business networks spanning the globe today, nodes and networks have been used in a number of psychological applications. An example of this is the concept of Semantic Differentials, the use of which having been enhanced greatly by Subjective Probability and Information Theory, together with General System theory.

The early use of Semantic Differentials was extremely primitive, but improved quantization and the weighting of (Peircean) signs in Semiotics, regarding contexts and themes in linguistic analysis, has made such usage quite a 'fine art'. It is now possible to conceive of an 'n-dimensional response *surface*' (see Appendix) being of great value.

Indeed, initial steps towards the uncovering of Truth by networks of supercomputers have been taken already – although not with this specific intention. The so-called *Semantic Web*, for instance, is being addressed in order to facilitate 'universal *meanings* ' for machines to read. As with machine understanding of the spoken word, there are deep and difficult waters ahead in tying down comprehension re contexts and themes (see Appendix).

The same considerations apply obviously to research and development in Artificial Intelligence and Robotics, but there seems to be nothing that cannot be overcome – given sufficient resources. It is worthy of note, however, that massive resistance will be encountered from many quarters.

In such areas, seminal work was undertaken in the 1980s (at ASWE), but it was nor reported openly in the Journal of Naval Science because of the retirement of the researcher (me). Internal reports remain (and have been accredited). A potentially 'pivotal' report was of an experiment that yielded results of statistical significance – experimental design, methodology, analysis, etc. are to be found in the Appendix and Bibliograhy.

The methodology involved the counting, weighting, and scoring of individual words as pointers to contexts pertaining to individual themes (e.g. the bipolar theme of 'Safety/Danger'. This could be done by a person or bya a computer program.

Examples are given in the report of computer applications in areas as diverse as politics, personnel selection, knowledge bases, communication centres, and artificial intelligence. Personal involvement is foreseeable in all psychology-based disciplines. Such analytical techniques are embodied in a simple program which can be enhanced and extended almost without limit.

It may be significant that this basic mechanism can, in principle, provide self-modification facilities for automatic adaptive systems – particularly in regard of systems akin to the so-called 'Semantic Web' or even military applications, such as drones and other craft. (see Truth; Warship Analogy).

OCKHAM'S RAZOR

The underlying philosophy of William of Ockham is shaky; but, to scientists and philosophers alike, it is helpful to have his 'Razor' always in mind. It runs: 'Entities are not to be multiplied beyond necessity' (see Blackburn, pp. 267-8). [in my opinion, it is a very great pity that Jung did not follow this particular advice – his views were, in some ways, consonant with the dictum, but in others they were quite the opposite]

Applications of the watchword are often along the lines of 'reductionistic' or 'nominalistic' lines, but they *do* have weaknesses (see Popper). However, the call for Simplicity is surely universal; and Platonism and Comprehensive Realism, supported by Process Philosophy, are fine examples of the limits to which Simplicity can be taken. [Mathematicians might call it 'Beauty']

OPERATING SYSTEMS

The operating system of a military warship has inclusions necessitated by its role and its real-time performance in a hostile environment safeguarding and nurturing Others. It, therefore, contains mechanisms for things peculiar to that environment, such as interrupting normal operations, cyclical introduction of programs and program suites, intercommunication with others, recovery from damage, driving weapon platforms and sensor platforms, avoiding self-harm, and so on.

The 'SUPERVISOR' is a huge suite of programs called in cyclically by the operating system (which runs its own 'computer time' for that purpose) to virtually 'run' the vessel. The supervisor has correspondingly huge powers, and these include the altering of priorities and resource availability. There are compelling operational reasons for this arrangement to obtain in military systems.

In particular, careful watch is kept on the amounts of time and other resources to be spent on monitoring and maintaining services to SELF (i.e. the system) and similar attentions given to OTHERs in the environment. Apart from this balance, the operations of Judgment and Perception (as seen by Jung) come under the sway of the Supervisor (but the allocation of these matters varies according to such things as system type functional requirements).

Every effort is made in the design of the operating system to minimize the input needed from the Command element – except, of course, emergency input – the purpose of which being to facilitate the easy transfer of authority to specialists and successive holders of the Command function. [This appears to mirror the drift in philosophy away from the ancient notion of an all-powerful commanding Self]

PASSIONS

Robert C. Solomon presents an outline of *'Emotions and the Meaning of Life'* in a form lending itself to mechanistic representation. He offers both an Analysis of emotions and a register of their Characteristic Features, thereby cross-linking with Ethel Spector Person and Rollo May, in particular.

Also cross-linked with all three authors given above are neurological reports on the neural bases of Truth, Beuty, Love, Empathy, etc., from (i) the Institute of Neurology, London (Times, 20/2/04) and (ii) reports in Times, 10/11/07. See Clynes on Sentics.

PLATONIC WORLD

A splendid description of Plato's world of mathematical forms is given by Roger Penrose in *Shadows of the Mind* (p. 412). It is too long to reproduce here, but it offers answers to many questions as to its contents. Worth quoting is the central fact of its existence, namely that this rests upon 'the profound, timeless, and nature of its concepts. Also, that their laws are 'independent of those who discover them' (p. 413). John Polkinghorne writes on the subject in the same vein, but he introduces religious dogma.

The list given by Penrose makes MacKay's notion of the mechanistic embodiment of a mathematical formula very plausible; and, likewise, consolidates ideas on the power of robotics – especially in the Platonic setting of affinitive search.

PLURALITY OF CONSCIOUSNESS

This is mentioned by Gordon Rattray Taylor in *The Natural History of the Mind*. The width of this acclaimed science-writer's knowledge is best indicated by a set of quotations, as follows [I have the author's permission to make them]:- '...consciousness is not thing but a graded series, and the series is distributed through graded structures. And when higher levels of consciousness are abolished by drugs or damage or self-inhibition, the lower levels remain functional' (p. 110). See, also, *Selves*; *Triune Brain*, etc.

'...Today Freud's rather imprecise idea – a mere description of behaviour – is seen to have a solid neurophysiological basis. This can even be demonstrated. In the few cases where both cerebral hemispheres have been removed in man, behaviour of this primitive type remains. And many aspects of schizophrenia can be accounted for in these terms' (p.111). See *Triune Brain...; Selves*.

'...I would expect emotions to overall patterns rather than to be produced by specific mechanisms, though it may be that the most basic emotions, such as rage and fear, established early in evolution, are produced by specific mechanisms and that only the higher emotions have an overall character' (p. 291). See, also, *Passions*; *'I'*; *Self*; etc.

'...The brain contains countless feedback loops, but the significant feature is that they are nested hypermorphically. Each level sets the aim for the level below...There are, then two contrasting brain systems: an analytic one which dissects the environment into units of information, and which works, so to say upwards, and an intentional one which

uses that information to affect the environment, and works, we may say, downward...'
(pp. 62-3).   See, also, *Encephalized Mind(Ego); Jungian Theory; Strong Dualistic Hypothesis; Attention;* etc.

PRIESTLEY

An entry in a Biographical Dictionary – over about three inches of column – describes J. B. Priestley as an 'astute, original and controversial commentator on contemporary society'.   His publishers, of *Man and Time*, use words like 'fascinating', 'delightful' and 'profound', and The New York Herald Tribune believes it to be one of hs most important books.

For me, it is *the* most important book, because it joins Jungian theory and Jungians of note with mathematics, mysticism, ESP, the workings of the brain/Mind(Ego), physics, and personal everyday kinds of experience.   He laces all these subjects together, and more, in an eminently readable 'package' and presents it to us with his best wishes.   His letter, asking for a copy of my putative book is one of my most cherished possessions.

PONTIFICAL NERVE-CELL

PRIMACY

Matter=   Negligible

Matter twinned with Spirit   =   Polkinghorne; Zohar

Spirit   =   Plato; Penrose; Motoyama;

PRINCIPLE

The under-pinning of a *conjectured* way of Being or Becoming that can be judged to exist or to obtain by virtue of apparently observed 'characteristics' or 'effects'.   The 'Reflection Principle', or 'Life Force', or 'Yin-Yan' are examples.   {Provided it is conjectured from a sound base, as these would be, a principle can be treated as a 'proposition' and, therefore, it can be awarded a quantitative value or degrees of belief (see Subjective Probability)}.

PRINCIPLE OF CONVERGENCE

PROCESS IMAGE/IDEAL FORM

PROCESS and PROCESS PHILOSOPHY

The mathematician and logician, A.N. Whitehead, devised the powerful theoretical system of thought called process philosophy in order to really 'get down to basics' – but it remains conjectural, although involving 'occasions of experience', events, and principles of concrescence and of limitation. Occasions of experience are events, but they cannot exist on their own.

They are, therefore, relational and they are arranged hierarchically with the largest and most complex groups being called 'societies'. Various principles of limitation govern the arrangement of growth up the hierarchy {this sounds rather reminiscent of Aristotle}.

Although solitary 'occasions' cannot exist (rather like magnetic monopoles) each occasion has two poles – one for mentation and one for persistence or endurance. These poles provide the occasion with what is called 'subjective aim' operating under the principle of concrescence or concretion.

It is postulated that there is nothing smaller than an occasion of experience [process philosophy was advanced before particle physics arrived on the scene] and this is exemplified often by statements that electrons are formed of occasions. The picture emerging from process philosophy is strikingly akin to processes in a computer system and in the Sino-Asiatic model.

PSYCHAGOGUES

Jung reports conversations with *psychagogues*, and by that term he was referring to a 'spirit guru'. That spirit guru, to which he referred under the name of *Philemon*, Jung saw to 'represent superior insight' (p.176). In his so called 'dream wanderings', Jung frequently encountered an old man accompanied by a young girl. He saw Salome as the companion of Elijah, and he comments that Salome is not only blind but is an also an Anima figure.

The coupling of the two, in a manner of speaking, brings together wisdom, intelligence, and knowledge. Salome's contribution to the relationship is of eroticism. These, stopping short of definition, might be regarded as *personifications* of the principles of *Logos* and of *Eros*. Today, there are Jungians, such as Timothy O'Neill, who would equate these features with *Yin* and and *Yang*, as sub-principles of the overall 'Life Force', issuing forth from the Spirit Body.

The Jung-Plato paradigm unifies all of this with experience and brings the whole system of thought into sharp focus. The Animus/Anima *is* the guide and guru of the individual woman/man towards *Re-union* in the Soul Body within the Spirit Body.

The Persona plays it part in the process. It can even be defined as that image of himself which 'Omar' would wish to be held by his Beloved. His goal would certainly be one of 'self-improvement' but *not* for himself. Any self-improvement would be aimed at improving either the lot of the Beloved or their relationship.

153

This brings Jungian theory into the category of Relationism (see the entry for it in this Part) and rationalizes it. It becomes *experiential* and it follows J.B. Priestley's words and experimental findings. Moreover, it squares with karma and rebirth in that *shared karma* is possible and the concepts of Williamson and Pearse concerning Health and 'Memory-Will' become upheld.

Of special importance is the fact that this promotes in the personality an outlook of complete 'openness' that contrasts so sharply with Jung's evaluation of Secrecy (p. 315) and the Self-knowledge that he advocates. Other things ensue, also, such as the use of 'soul-constant' to describe Penelope the wife of Odysseus, which points up the flaws in Jungian interpretation of the myth.

Laurens van der Post is the user of the term, and he describes Penelope as possibly the greatest 'personification of the soul constant in man provided he endures to the true end in his search to rejoin her'(p. 164). This is unexceptional. What *is* exceptional is his linking this with the 'balderdash' (see Munroe) that represents the misconception of 'internal completion' through much taradiddle about the growth of the Animus/Anima and its being discarded after this 'completion'

The 'taradiddle' reaches absurdity when van der Post (p. 234) not only to 'four self-evident ascending' models': Eve, Helen of Troy, Mary, and Sophia (not my choice by any means), but also tofour corresponding to support his own achievements in Lao-Tzu, Mani, Buddha and Christ. No comment is needed.

In comparing all this with the proposed Jung-Plato paradigm, William of Ockham would surely have been almost overwhelmed by the beautiful simplicity of the proposal. [The term 'beatiful' is commonly used by mathematicians and physicists to describe features – as is the term 'elegant']

QUATERNIONS

The dictionary definition of a quaternion is: four similar elements, with one element being different in some fundamental way from the others. Jung chose to illustrate this by way of charting the growth of the Animus/Anima (*not* of Love) from the symbol Eve, through those of Helen and Mary, to *Sapientia*. [a very odd ragbag of symbols].

In that quaternion, however, there *does* appear to be a possible *transition point* from a triage of awareness and identity and something transcendent (outside the physical universe) or something ethereal (in the Penrose sense), or something transcendental and exact copied into the imperfect ethereal. This, as in the warship, is on the premise that the transcendental form is inaccessible to inferior entities.

Such a situation could obtain from a triune brain and/or a plurality of consciousness, and/or a declension in the power and range of a succession of identities.

The are many incomplete versions of an arrangement of this kind.   But, the classical Greeks seem to have perceived some similar progression in going from *body*, through the processing of information by a mind (thymos), to the soul (psyche) – see Joan Wynn Reeves.

QUARTIC ORGANUM

We can discuss 'consciousness' from very first principles to the latest analysis conducted by the acclaimed and serious science writer, Rita Carter. Although this process is related by her only to unitary consciousness' (in terms of brain functions) as distinct from what has been called 'plurality of consciousness', it suffices for my purposes in regard of 'mystical experience'.

Following biological evolution, we start with a single-cellular creature reacting to stimuli as though distinguishing between 'self' and 'other'. And, starting from set theory, we start with a notion of 'nothing' that can only be represented numerically by the use of 'something', i.e. a set. This has considerable significance for the endorsement and segmentation of the 'Axis of Scale' and 'hidden dimensions'; and the roots of set theory, and the roots of set theory are very much our business.

Much further along the evolutionary trail, a quaternion can be discerned that has three elements of Judgment relating to 'self' and the fourth element pertaining to 'other'. All the elements are types of relationship, and the same functions of Judgment and Perception are present whether the organism performing the judgment and perception is living or non-living.

This translates into activities of thought, or of reasoning, or of learning (i.e. of acquiring knowledge). This process was first envisaged by Aristotle (deduction). It was augmented by Bacon (induction), and then it was carried further by Ouspensky (*intuition*). We can complete the quaternion (of means of gaining knowledge) with mystical experience.

The set of four is a quaternion because the first three organa are means of deriving or securing knowledge, whereas the fourth is from the *mystical experience* of sharing it – either from indwelling, or from union, or from merger.   Each of these is different. William Johnston provides both the order and a discussion]

Rita Carter states that 'every type of seeming-spiritual experience could be explained' by the actions of material neurons (p. 290).   She proceeds to ask whether spiritual experience (of transcendence) is merely an aberration of consciousness.   She, then, remarks how difficult it is to dismiss intuitive logic once you have experienced it. But, Ms Carter has here mixed categories twice.

She has confused intuition with *sharing of experience*; and she has confused the *material* with the *physical*.   She has not heeded the recognized distinction between *mysticism* and *religious mysticism*.   The two are quite different from each other.   The former relates to non-material functions within the physical universe, and it is the latter which is transcendental. Knowledge obtained by mystical experience (quartic organum) is undeniable.

QUINTIC ORGANUM

If the 'soul' and its 'ideal form' exist, then we can define *quartic* organum as the means (organ) by which knowledge is gained jointly and simultaneously (through experience) by the equal and opposite 'poles' of a spiritual entity in the physical world. Quintic organum would, then, be definable as the onwards transmission of that knowledge (in 'twinned' perspective and, therefore, 'improved') from the ideal form to the 'User'

This notion is not too discordant with many schemes of thought in which 'dialogue' is held between individuals and their God(s). In terms of very densely packed data compression it can even be sensed. However, it *does* pose a number of theological and philosophical questions about possible attenuation, or misrepresentation, etc., and, in such a case, William of Ockham might have said: Do not multiply interfaces without necessity.

Thoughts, such as these, are not absent from any critical review of hierarchical 'progression' or 'ascension'. And, they are applicable, also, to Jung's notion of man beingraised from the animals by his reflective power so as to develop and spread 'meaning' – which is dubious, anyway.

RANK

Otto Rank, as did Jung, conceived Libido as very much grander and more majestically powerful, than Freud's concept. He came to Psychotherapy from outside psychology – from engineering – and some might consider that an advantage. He focussed primarily upon the (constructive) Will, which he conceived as, *by its nature*, a relationship with the 'other' (Munroe, p. 591)

As (i) Smolin considers the whole universe to be nothing but relationships and fields, (ii) the natural quaternion organizes and constrains biological relationships, (iii) the social Leviathan feeds upon relationships, (iv) Sherrington sees Nature's Aim as all relationships being altruistic, (v) Rollo May sees polarized relationships as being ontologically necessary, (vi) Systems Methodology sees Polarity as a metaphysical assumption, and (vii) existential love has its roots in matter but goes beyond physical, emotional, and erotic love, it does seem that Otto Rank might just have been 'on to something' (!?).

And so, we find in today's society that 'talking about sex is is the easiest way of avoiding really making any *decisions* about love and sexual relatedness' (May, p. 196). I would add to this the reflection that it (talking about sex) is also, in many ways, part of the social Leviathan's armoury. Few people in today's world would deny Jung's assertion that Evil is determinant reality.

All of these things point up Otto Rank's belief that the 'will orientation of the person' is the key issue of mental health (Munroe, p. 579) and that the mature person loves himself in the other, and the other in himself (p. 584). They all point towards the key Jungian orientation choice between Self and Other.

REFLECTION PRINCIPLE

RELATIONAL HOLISM

Holistic Relationism is a better term for describing a world consisting of only relations and fields than 'relational holism' because it introduces more necessary elements, such as normative and deontic features. For example, it brings in notions of 'hierarchical nesting' and the ordering of goals by priorities. It is, therefore, concomitant with the idea of Comprehensive Reality and the warship paradigm, in which the whole organism exhibits those characteristics. (see Holistic Relationism)

RELATIONISM

In regard of this subject, there has been a drift in Philosophy away from its use in natural language which, in my opinion, introduces a certain loss of accuracy in communication. Both the *Shorter Oxford English Dictionary* (SOED) and the *Chambers Dictionary* give essentially the same definitions, but I have found no dictionary of philosophy which contains it.

The definition is twofold. (a) the doctrine of the relativity of knowledge and (b) the doctrines that relations have a real existence. Clearly, the thesis in this monograph includes both concepts.

RIEMANNIAN GEOMETRY

For this monograph, it suffices to know that this geometry describes 'higher-level' analogues of curved surfaces, and that the Riemannian zeta function is a function of a complex variable that is associated with Roger Penrose's twistor theory.

His book, *The Road to Reality*, is aimed at being 'A Complete Guide to the Physical Universe' and, so far a I can understand it, it completes that mission. For a layman in mathematics, like myself, it is jam-packed with very useful diagrams; and the one most pertinent to this entry is on page 135 (Fig, 8.1) and shows how the Riemannian surface for log z is a 'spiral ramp flattened down vertically to the complex plane'.

Readers may remember that 'plausibility' is log odds, which can be derived from the logistic function, and that I indicate the complex plane in relation to the Sino-Asiatic model in my Figure 2.   This appears to be consonant with the remark, made by Penrose, that mathematical representation of duality is a matter for elsewhere.

ROBOTICS and COMPUTATION

In the same way that physicists appear sometimes drawn along a blind alley in their thinking, so neuroscientists and mathematicians seem to become pre-occupied or side-tracked by false leads.   They seem sometimes, for example, to think that things achieved by neural networks should be achievable at the level of individual neurons. This hardy seems logical.

Although it was being pointed out fifty years ago that individual neurons should be treated as mini- computers, many individual features of the human brain contribute to its Judgment and perception, and this is reflected in Sherrington's 'principle of convergence' and in MacKay's 'mechanistic embodiment', and many other features from Artificial Intelligence (AI).

As a consequence, many man-hours of effort have been wasted, it seems to me, on 'computability' – especially on the ideas of Alan Turing, the originator of the 'Turing Test'. This test was to see whether a computer (i.e. a program suite) could pass as a human being. Even then it was possible to do so by intruding 'stalling' mechanisms of the kind so prevalent in the human - 'You know'.

I suppose this capacity to be shared with the Anima/animus, and with Defence Mechanisms, in Jungian terms.   But these facilities introduce a different category into the term 'computability'.   Alternatively, it could be labelled as 'Protective Mimicry' – a characteristic of Evolution and of heuristic learning, relational databases, and Semiotics.

An interesting point, in this regard, concerns robots. I have often suggested, in principle, that robots could conduct a search for their particular 'elective affinity' if they were given some simple number as a starting point and homing point, [This is merely an extension of the Turing test].

Rudy Rucker makes a similar point in *INFINITY & THE MIND* (p.186). He does so in reference to the kind of phenomenon – non-locality – that is conjectured to obtain in living cells. Rucker suggests that, if 'entanglement' of particles is true, one might choose to identify one's mind with the cosmos rather than with some individual brain.   In the Jung-Plato paradigm we have opportunities for both to obtain (in a universe of hierarchical nesting.

Rudy Rucker points out that 'there is no reason why such a form of higher consciousness would not be open to robots as well.   This rather depends upon the possibility that matter is infinitely divisible; and he refers back to Cantor's remark that 'the infinite even inhabits our minds'.

SELF

One of the descriptions given by Jung (1964, pp. 354-5) of the Self is: '…the totality of the personality…'; and, elsewhere, in the same volume (p. 197) he declares that his whole life has been 'permeated and held together' by one idea and one goal, i.e. to penetrate into the 'secret of the personality'. In another place (p. 188) he tells us that 'the goal of psychic development is the self'.

The so-called Jungian 'problematic' features the distinction between 'Self' and 'Other', and in the volume, *Jung in Modern Perspective*, it is repeated and consolidated that Jungian theory comes down on the side of 'Self'. The composition and dissociation of the psyche is fixed solidly upon 'the secret of Personality'. However, this situation appears to be utterly erroneous.

I say this because each and every one of the characteristic and typical features associated by Jung with Personality turns out to be equally applicable to a *real-time computer system* and hence to a hypothesized *mental* system. They describe an encephalized 'mind' and its identities. The Freudian concepts of *id, Ego,* and *Superego* suffice to explain them as the software of the brain's hardware, and thus to provide Personality for the Mind(Ego) by way of neural circuits.

This dissolves the whole underpinning of the Self and the psyche. Any remnant of Jung's concept of the psyche is reduced to that which was conjectured by the Greeks of the time of Plato and Aristotle, namely as a Command element giving assent or dissent to actions proposed by the Mind(Ego). And, this squares with modern thought outside the Jungian opus.

It is consonant with Sherrington's 'ultimate, pontifical nerve-cell', and with Priestley's Self 3, and with the 'inner Self' pictured by Popper and Eccles, and with the 'causal' self of the Motoyama model, and with the system envisaged by William James which issues the Command fiat from the 'superconscious', and even with an etherealized ideal form (see Penrose). So, the notion of a non-material Command element cannot yet be written off.

Former Jungians (e.g. Jolande Yacobi; M.-L. von Franz) and modern ones (e.g. T. O'Neill) have shown Jungian theory to be consonant with particle physics and Hinduism from certain perspectives. Contrasting the two former with the latter throws clear cut light on the Animus/Anima. Experience is written in also by Sherrington, Ethel Person, Rollo May, Alister Hardy, and numerous others; and Whitehead's theoretical process philosophy makes a wonderful sounding board for ideas in that respect (see process philosophy).

SELF-DISCOVERY

Jung impressed upon us the need for self-analysis – rigorous, deep, sparing nothing – *if we want to understand the problem of evil* (my italics). He asserted that man was raised from the animals by his *power of reflection* (italics inserted). Why, then, did he fail to suggest the immense and necessary power of 'reflective self-discovery?

Several possible answers come to mind – the question is not a rhetorical one. The most obvious one is, perhaps, that unconsciously he did not dare to really discover his true nature – this is a possibility, in view of his personal life (that he wanted, also, to keep 'private').

He was motivated, too, by his desire to be 'better' than Freud; and he was justified in this by his postulation of dualism between matter and non-matter (but being wrong in the detail). The most likely reason is a compounded one of these two reasons taking into account, as a whole, his nature, nurture, and circumstances (leaving his deep 'inner self' unknown and, perhaps, unknowable).

Such impressions are not negated by Jung's statement (p. 191) that everything important in his theory has held good since his student days and everything after that has been a refinement of those central features. 'Inner self' is an expression used by Popper and Eccles that approaches close to the nature of Jung's concept of the psyche once the 'mind(Ego)' has been encephalized.

SELVES

Common Sense, Information Mechanics, and Experience, all argue for the existence of Sherrington's 'ultimate pontifical (psychical) nerve-cell' in which 'brain' collaborates with 'psyche'. It can be argued that the psychical aspect of the 'nerve-cell' is in some dimension(s) of the physical universe that is 'beyond' the senses and perceptions of our everyday life. Indeed, the thought of transfinite 'atoms' permeating his brain-cells did nothing to help Cantor's mental health.

It may be that Taxonomy is a felicitous subject from which to approach the bewildering variety of entities and identities that faces us: I have to break it down structurally to explain them. Therefore, I put forward a triage of identities nominated Self 1, Self 2, and Self 3 (after Priestley). And, as we encounter each, I will cross-reference them to other entries in this Glossary.

Self 1 is J.B. Priestley's basal identity which experiences pain or discomfort. It says to itself (metaphorically) 'there is pain'. However, it is probably a collection of neurons at the level of the brain stem and limbic system functioning as the reptilian brain while also stretching out laterally – following the brain's evolution – to serve as the self-adjusting *operating system* for the evolving mammalian and human brains, i.e. Brain/Mind(Ego).

We may surmise, from the *taxonomy* of system types, that the difference between real and artificial, i.e. real-time *computer systems,* is indeterminate and moving all the time towards the artificial. Furthermore, that the mechanisms of Self 1 are capable of discerning between *Self* and 'Other'. Hence, the notion arises of Extraversion and

Introversion in both the living system and the non-living system, and the occurrence of the same kind of distinction being made at the level of protozoans (see Roger Penrose).

Self 2 in the 'Priestley – Bennett - Ouspensky' model is the forecasting of consequential events based upon the experience of Self 1   The idea arises: 'I will feel more pain'.   There seems to be no reason for supposing that this cannot be by heuristic learning coupled with the parallel evolution of relational and associative memories by way of the understanding of signs (see Elizabeth Bates).

All of this is well within the capabilities of a *warship's real-time computer system* under its Commander.   At times, and under certain circumstances, the vessel *per se* runs autonomously.   However, for most operational situations a human Command element is necessary to give the final assent or dissent for the computer's proposed actions.

Self 3, in the same model (Priestley – Bennett - Ouspensky), is the entity which says to itself, Well, I shall soon perceive Self 1 and Self 2 learning about pain.   The wording is not an exact quotation but it suffices - the differentiation is clear.   This declension or *triage* corresponds very closely to the Classical Greeks identification of body, knowledge-processing (thymos) associated with the body, and the Psyche (commonly associated today with the '*soul*').

If we take the most severe case of determinism that we can think of, which is presented in this book, there is always a situation in which Self 1 and Self 2 are mechanistically embodied and some entity outside the body gives the Command fiat. According to Donald MacKay, this is from the 'ideal form', i.e. the embodied formula, which can always be *different from what it is.*

The difficulty with this is the enclosure of the ideal form within God.   This is the only thing about which we disagreed – I maintained that the ideal form should be additionally 'free-standing' and along the lines of the Penrosean 'etheriality'. Mathematical Platonism seems to avoid even that element of choice, but it still provides a choice of adhering to one's 'story' or not doing so.   If there were no choice at all, an organism would be merely an automaton.

The triage of 'Selves' fits admirably with Ouspensky's notions and with the large number of respondents to Priestley's television request for reports upon 'psychical' experiences from viewers.   It fits equally well with evolutionary psychology – except for the puzzling persistence of choice and/or free will.   Even MacKay's *Comprehensive Realism* cannot eliminate that.

SAPIENTIA

Sapientia, in natural language, is defined in terms of Sapience, as: Wisdom, Understanding, Correct taste and judgment, *or* used depreciatively or ironically: would-be wisdom (SOED).   It is difficult to find the name, Sapientia, anywhere other than in traditional Jungian literature or (once) in mystical texts pertaining to the 'journey of love' (Johnston, 1981, p.139).

William Johnston refers to *growth* from the erotic to the mystical depicted by Jung symbolically as Eve (biological love), Helen of Troy, the Virgin Mary (devotional love), and Sapientia or Wisdom (mystical love). Johnston goes on, to say: The idea of Jung is that, ideally speaking, human love should grow and develop through these stages – though he admits that in our day very few people reach the fourth and mystical stage.

Now, here, I feel inclined to say something like 'if only' and then go on to point out that reading and re-reading Jung reveals a complete contrast. Jung re-asserted his beliefs in *Memories, Dreams, Reflections* (and particularly in its Glossary). *My* repeated reading of Jung is of the condemnation of emotional ties (despite the natural quaternion); of that quaternion of symbols); of the symbolic progression being of the growth of the Animus/Anima (in *Man and his Symbols*); and of the goal of psychic development being the Self.

I agree (almost) entirely with William Johnston's interpretation – but that is not what Jung said. Jung could not, or would not, make *experience* central to his theory – despite his fine words on the pre-eminence of Experience. Neither could he promote personal love because of his involved and strange relationships with women in his private and personal life.

His long paragraph on cosmogonic love has him delegating love to God, but even that introduces all kinds of attributions to love that surely are unjustified. Despite his fine words to certain ladies about their being *femmes inspiratrices'* it seems most unlikely that he ever experienced or encountered Sapientia. (see MYSTICISM etc.; INDIVIDUATION; COLLECTIVE UNCONSCIOUS)

SET THEORY

A *set* is 'any collection of things or numbers that belong to a well-defined *category'*. There are several ways of describing a set, including natural language descriptions and mathematical ones. As the latter rests upon sounder foundations, it would seem that definitions of this type are to be preferred.

The former type, i.e. natural language, rests upon the powers of human ratiocination to assign features under consideration to *categories*, and Ludwig von Bertalanffy discusses this (see *General System Theory*). This is fallible (see APPENDIX). However, Categorization can play an important part in Psychological Analysis, so a clear distinction may be made between *Mathematical Analysis* and *Psychological Analysis*.

SEX AND LOVE

Sex and Love may seem to be at opposite ends of a *hierarchy* despite many limbs of the social Leviathan arguing that they are the same thing. If we go back in Evolution to the association of *Learning and Emotion* pictured by Livesey we find, almost *ab initio,* that the process of Heuristic Learning is associated with Emotion.

This begs the question: '*Are* Sex and Love two sides of the same coin?' To dualists and pluralists the question seems rhetorical, and Artificial Intelligence supports their rhetoric because the finest real-time systems that exist are intelligent enough but they are, nevertheless, _Support_ systems for a User or Users.

The User may not prove to be as Jung and others of the same inclination would like but in the manifestations of the spirit in the material world it seems true. For example, we are told that the male interest in sexual activities last almost twice as long as a woman's, and this is consonant with the drive of Evolution for survival of the species.

But survival of the species has little to do with Love. So, can Love arise from the coupling (pun intended) of Emotion and Learning? Even if we go really hard-line to *Robotics* we find that a completely life-like robot could easily satisfy Turing's Test (passing successfully as a human) but it could never partake in a heuristic search for the other part of its soul (but see Rucker).

Unless, that is, the Creator (us) gave it some unique identifier to allow the discovery to be made. Williamson and Pearse identified this matching as being like a key fitting into a lock, but that would not necessarily be unique – unless we had created lots of robotic pairs, each very slightly different from the other. This would not only fit with our experience but would gel with mathematical Platonism.

We would also see that the enjoyment of sex is vastly different from the delight, nay bliss, arising from the implanted motivation. And, there are many other equal gradings of enjoyment, in sport, in scholarship, in many, many kinds of activities non-related to Sex.

The sex drive in the material world of Nature is (or can be) extremely strong and it can shade our Judgment and Perception. Jung was clearly wrong in urging us to exclude all emotional 'ties' (the term indicates his attitude). Emotion is keyed into Learning, and Learning includes recognition of *bonds* with Parents, Offspring, Siblings, and Others. The social Leviathan uses the bonds to snare its victims, but they _are_ existents and must be addressed.

The sex drive is part of the Charioteer's (Plato's simile) Black Horse. Plato advised that the black horse should be *controlled* by the Charioteer, not 'put down'. It is (can be) so strong that each individual is forced to deal with it in his/her own way.

Jung was quite correct over this aspect of Life in his insistence upon conflicts of interest. Freud was correct, also, in *his* insistence upon the power of the Sex Drive. *He* introduced the concepts of Conscience and of the Superego (two different phenomena).

Rollo May, in *Love and Will*, maintains that both Sex and Love are necessary to shape our actions. Many people in our society today lament the blurring of distinctions between the two. Indeed, C.S. Lewis, the Christian apologist, depicted in *That Hideous Strength* how humans had perfected means of enjoying sexual pleasure utterly divorced from procreative intent (Barbarella's 'Exquisite Pleasure Machine' comes to mind!?).

Sex, in particular, is an area in which common sense does NOT seem to abound. For example, cases of mothers fixing prophylactic patches on their daughters at a very young age because 'they're bound to have sex' is somewhat dubious. And, on finding condoms in their young daughter's handbag, refraining from giving her prophylactic patches in the belief that 'it is too early'. These are sociological problems that are faced by Welfare Officers daily – and who would have their job?

In these cases, there are labyrinthine networks of muddled thinking *and* exploitation at work. There is 'grooming', for example, and sometimes jealousy. Sometimes it feels sensible to remove children and sometimes this proves to be correct. At other times it proves to be wrong. There is always, it seems, someone to champion the actions of a clear miscreant.

And, much the same can be said about Love. Jung's tirade about Eros, for example, is embarrassing. Having decried the vicissitudes brought about by 'emotional ties' in the first place, he picks on Eros for taking us at times to the depths of Hell, and then 'boots the ball into the long grass' by identifying God as 'Cosmogonic Love'.

SOUL

There is sometimes confusion between the terms 'soul' and 'spirit', especially concerning their primacy and the relation between them, but W.E.R. Mons, in *Beyond Mind*, gives us clear definitions. He indicates the relationship between them in terms of both function and of relative positions.

Both 'soul' and 'spirit' have close associations with Christianity, but Mons is a psychiatrist of wide experience and very great clarity of thought (and expression), and he conceives of a *Spirit God of Psychic Power* (p. 230). His conception is similar to Teilhard's notion of a universal spread of 'perfected souls'.

His book is one that warrants interest as a primer and/or source-book because it covers a perspective from psychiatry, on psychiatry, from Victorian times up to its publication. In a sense, it is a companion for the work by Guy Lyon Playfair over the same period. Their titles give a suggestion of this in *Beyond Mind* (Mons) and *The Indefinite Boundary* (Playfair)

Beyond Mind includes reference to Gurdjieff, Ouspensky, Nicol, and Bennett, and others, who (apart from Gurdjieff) went on to develop independent schools of psycho-philosophy (p. 200).

It is from Mons that we learn of the juxtapositioning of soul and spirit (p. 194). He quotes Steiner:

The spirit is the central point of man, the body the intermediary by which the spirit observes and learns to understand the physical world and through which man acts in it. The soul is the intermediary between the two.

Walter Mons, on the same page, then outlines the Church's supposed (at the time) or believed constituents of man:

1. The familiar physical body

2. A semi-physical vital body or 'vehicle of vitality' which animates it

3. A super-physical Soul-Body which uses these two

4. A true, transcendental Spirit-Body, a formless radiation rarely if ever perceived.

Sometimes, a simple dichotomy between 'physical' (I.e. of the physical universe) and 'transcendental' is sufficient. An alternative is to distinguish between Matter and Non-Matter – depending on the context. Another alternative is to follow Williamson and Pearse in coining a different vocabulary, but that might be to introduce complications. See Spirit, Superconscious, Strong Dualistic Hypothesis.

Other examples of the book's usefulness are the reference to Jung's not making *experience* central to his theories and the remark that Jung brought Plato's ideas up-to-date. However, Mons does not refer to mathematics, or to mathematical Platonism, or to Alfred North Whitehead, or to teleology – hence my earlier comments. The scheme produced by Mons is of evolutionary emergence which is not enough.

Another tinge of early days is the focus upon 'radiations', however we must bear in mind that Plato writes of moving shadows projected through a fire on to a cave wall. Furthermore, we talk frequently today of 'cosmic' radiation, and Mons, himself, mentions St. Paul and his seeing through a glass, darkly. Another simile, which might be preferable to some, is the colourful rays of sunshine that come through the stained glass windows of a church or cathedral.

The last two similes can be accompanied by a third one that is applicable to the Jung-Plato paradigm. The notion of Life *Energy* passing through the regime of mathematics and ending up as living material entities, in essence, is not unlike those two. Furthermore, the MacKay model (of 'mechanistic embodiment' in a system of Comprehensive Reality) is a worthy contender for a fourth parallel simile.

Moreover, the scheme would equate the soul with an 'Ideal Form' or 'Specification', and the flow of information would be the same. A discrepancy, in this case, would be that MacKay, on the one hand, equated the 'implemented' entity with a mathematical formula but, on the other hand, believed that there is no need for ideal forms as the 'formula' is held in the mind of God.

It is not inconceivable that the 'Higgs boson' may one day be found to play a part in the channelling of information in the similes given above that feature Radiation. The *nadis* and *chakras* of the Hindu yogic tradition feature energy and the transmission of energy (see Motoyama, p. 11).

SPIN

SPIN – a simple 'four-letter word' that plunges one immediately into the deepest (and darkest) depths of philosophy (and cosmology). It is argued that the physical universe is composed only of relationships and fields, but clearly one can go 'deeper' than this. Relationships are between entities, for example, and process philosophy (and Religion, and Mathematical Platonism, and Comprehensive Realism, and Hinduism) takes us into unknown (but experiential) Realms in which the only existents are (it seems) solely energy and spin.

This notion can be exemplified by reference to the Axis of Scale. As we go towards the positive Transfinite, so we encounter (all within the same volume of traditional space-time) Realm One which is compose of atoms and molecules. Realm Two contains the smaller Fermions and Bosons distinguished only by their spin (in terms of Planck units of measurement), and Realm Three contains only Leptons and Quarks (and ephemeral sub-particles).

Electrons are interesting little creatures for they all have the same kind of spin. Except, that is, when they come under the influence of magnetic fields. I say 'creatures' following the examples of John Polkinghorne, who sees them as Real, and A.N. Whitehead, who sees them as being composed of 'occasions of experience'.

Currently, however, occasions of experience (seen as 'events') may not obtain everywhere and everywhen, because before the beginning (i.e. the hypothesized Big-Bang) there was no Time or Space —only energy and spin. This squares with Polkinghorne's concept of the 'domain of the Big-Bang', and with Platonism. It is consonant also with the Hindu yogic tradition (see Motoyama and Johnston).

SPIRIT

A glance at any reputable dictionary indicates a bewildering variety of meanings for the term 'spirit'. One is forced, therefore, to set one's own preferred (and reasoned) definition and then to elaborate, if required, on versions of it. So, it seems reasonable to set a fairly loose definition to start with and the to harden it up during the process.

Despite the term 'spirit' invoking a range of concepts from Biblical to Victorian at its worst (e.g. Spiritualism and Spiritism), the term *does* have intuitive but sensible meanings that are virtually universal. So, in a universe consisting of only relationships and 'fields', I must overcome my reluctance and talk (acceptingly) of Spirit as if it were a 'substantial entity' when in reality the term 'substantial' is completely inappropriate.

It is, in truth, the medium through which forces flow so as to produce a *manifestation* of substance. For example, in the physical Realm, the Life Force (of the so-called Spirit Body) frees the Yin and Yang to 'arrange' the manifestation of male and female bodies [as I understand Motoyama]. The notion of 'Principle's operating in this way is conconant with process philosophy.

The *spirit body* is also an entity that can issue or direct forces such as the Yin and the Yang, and the Life Force. It is a User of Energy and a Provider of Energy. It is also a Director of Energy Flow. it is not a material entity, although one feels it should have some kind of Personalty.

And, although the idea may seem to some 'fanciful' to some, I feel that it is their objections which are flimsy and unsustainable.   In short, there is no spirit 'Realm', as such, spirit is everywhere .   It is present all along the Axis of Scale, for example.   Such things (entities) as 'souls' and 'psyches' are 'arrangements' of Whitehead's 'occasions of experience'.

Guy Lyon Playfair once used the term '*The Indefinite Boundary*' to describe the zone between the physical world and the spiritual world.   Although today we think more in terms of dimensions or scale, Playfair's term is still useful.   To me, it brings up a picture of a zone or realm or Realm 'somewhere' along the axis of scale between the Planck limits of space and of time and the world of mathematical Platonism.   Thus, it includes, in order, Laszlo's 'extra' level in the quantum vacuum and the 'ethereality' level of Roger Penrose.

STRONG DUALISTIC HYPOTHESIS

SUBJECTIVE PROBABILITY

Following the ideas of the Reverend Thomas Bayes, much earlier, I.J. Good devised a measure of uncertainty which he called, *plausibility*, and which could be awarded *degrees of belief* in *quantitative* terms which could be added together so as to produce a *weight of evidence*.   This was for individual Judgment, but there is no apparent reason why (under terms and conditions) why the measures cannot be extended into group-judgment.

A decade or so later, unknowingly, I devised the same measure of uncertainty, i. e. plausibility, to simplify and improve processes in radar probability theory.   I derived it, however, from a common growth function (the logistic) because I suspected it would be useful in terms of information growth in those matters (it turned out to be useful in many other fields of interest).

It seems, consequently, that I happened to tie subjective probability into information theory – thereby infusing the latter with the virtues of the former and consolidating both.   The fundamental notion is that conjectural 'propositions' can be given numerical weightings which can be accumulated, provided that the propositions are formulated on a 'sound' body of beliefs.

Naturally, I put this concept to the test experimentally – using an experimental design that used six people (three men and three women) over ten trials and asking them to simulate, as best they could, the 'reptilian' faculties in their brain to evaluate the separate and distinct reports given in standard texts and using words as 'signs' (indexes of the Peircean kind –see Bates).   The results showed that a number of factors were statistically significant and worthy of note.

From Information theory, the story moves on to set theory and other mathematical affairs, discussed primarily by Roger Penrose in sixty three pages on 'Truth, Proof, and Insight' in *The Emperor's New Mind* (1990, pp. 129-193).   Rudy Rucker, likewise, addresses set theory in *'Infinity and the Mind'*. Daintith and Rennie even refer to the fascinating subject of 'transfinite induction' (p.221).

Perhaps more significant, however, is that – some sixty-five years after Good's 'landmark in the statistical reawakening of Bayesian theory' (Savage, p 10) – Bayesian theory is being mooted in Academia (Cornell University avoids all the uncertainties of quantum theory by using measures of Likelihood).

SUBORDINACY and SUPERORDINATION

Subordination

Jung appears to have phrased it well when he wrote of man being raised from 'mere being' by his reflective powers, but a moment's reflection reveals that, yet again, he sounds good but is wrong. The whole of the animal kingdom – of which man is a part – cannot be discarded as 'mere being'.

Disregarding that aside, we reflect that Man, in due course, conceived of pagan gods of various kinds, and then he began to feel pressures (or pulls) within himself (from a huge number of supposed sources including religions that are more organized – either Revealed or otherwise).

Donald MacKay would have phrased this, no doubt, as man feeling the need for divine Grace. And it would have been received in the 'core of the organism's self-organizing machinery', or its accessories, such as its 'priority ordering matrices'.

David Stafford-Clarke, God-fearing Freudian psychiatrist, has already pointed out that even after long and successful clinical treatment an individual is left with only his own powers. If that individual cannot cope with the stresses and strains of normal life, then Stafford-Clarke recommended Christianity.

Today, thoughts come to mind not of 'God slots', but of 'God spots' in the brain and 'User input'. Or, of ultimate supreme pontifical nerve-cells. And, the fact always remains that the 'brain/mind(Ego) is so *significantly* like a real-time 'Intelligent Support System' that it should be categorized as such. See Taxonomy.

The individual items of this Guide possess, in a considerable number of cases, inherent feelings of 'something' higher than the conscious Ego that has *superordinacy* but not completely so. Jung found this more difficult to encapsulate than was necessary because, we should remember, he ascribed the conscious ego to the non-material psyche.

The encephalization of the mind(Ego) resolves that difficulty and endorses what is implied in Jung's comment, namely 'evolutionary psychology' and the 'comprehensive reality' described by Donald MacKay. Jung's other remarks on this topic are appropriate and, it seems, they reflect a common phenomena – that of feeling 'in dialogue' with some entity that may be 'higher' but is not autocratic.

This entity is felt by many and it is given various names, some of which are more indicative than others of the nature of the entity. The 'entity' *does* seem to be an internal subsystem of the 'organism' – hence Sherrington's nomination of a supreme 'ultimate pontifical nerve cell'. But, Sherrington *does* describe how 'brain collaborates with Psyche'.

Likewise, Popper and Eccles describe *The Self and Its Brain*, the striking feature of which is what they call, 'the inner self'. Although the authors identify this 'inner self' with the 'soul' and the 'Self', they also identify it with the Ego, whichsays much about their dubious decision to avoid psychology and religion.

Freud came quite close to capturing this elusive inner self when he discriminated between Superego and Conscience, but this does not convey the *fact* that the Ego has the ability to pursue its own purposeful way despite the strong, almost *tangible* 'disapproval' and cautionary 'pressure' of this subsystem.

A former archbishop, in his book on *Mysticism in Religion* remarks that when he prays, miracles happen. When he prays, they *do* happen. And, a most moving message – in the St. Valentine's Day messages in a leading newspaper – which is impressed on my mind is: 'Where there is great love, miracles happen'. What a story must lie behind that! I hope very much that there was a happy ending for the lovers, and that no pain was suffered by anyone.

Returning more directly to the point. Jung found that he could deal successfully with this kind of 'dialogue' by following the feelings that he was given by his adviser. After a somewhat rocky start, I found that *my* adviser could be almost 'calibrated' by its 'success rate', and so I followed suit. As did Jung, I 'know' that the advice is sound.

Popper and Eccles conceived of two kinds of 'input' to the brain. One is a kind of standard procedure whereby the input undergoes a series of processing (primary, secondary, and tertiary) to ensure its 'soundness'. The other is for emergencies only whereby this processing is waived to save time. Special Purpose 'buttons' are pressed to enable this.

We conjecture that their proposition is sound because exactly the same procedure is used in the warship's computer driven 'Intelligent Support System'. Hence, it can be assumed that Sherrington's 'ultimate pontifical nerve cell' makes use of these forms, and that the Animus/Anima (in the Jung-Plato paradigm) can do likewise (in a more oblique or tangential way).

There are other ways of input, however, which are less clear-cut and less secure. I refer to what are called 'Service Streams', which do exactly as their title suggests, and by 'data links'. There are other phenomena, such as 'data-chaining' to save space, but these are more appropriate to other topics.

Service streams are (were, in my day) notoriously 'tricky'. Get the invoking protocol wrong and one is in 'big trouble'. Imagine the Sorcerer's Apprentice. Data links were highly classified at one time, but today they are multifarious and 'to be expected' as a 'matter of course'.

This package of measures from the fields of information transmission and communication (which is applicable to - and operative within - hierarchies of groups of warships), corresponds extremely closely to Jung's notion of a personal unconscious, a racial unconscious, and a collective unconscious.

Although the intermediate level is often omitted these days (undoubtedly for political correctness) it still holds good. Indeed, my ideas on this topic have been checked at high level with Jungians and have been met with approval and some enthusiasm.

It accords with the Hindu yogic tradition as its structures and functions are outlined by Motoyama and, also, with the appreciation of Mysticism and Buddhism as it is described By William Johnston. It brings into focus the way in which Jung tampered with the I Ching, as is evidenced in *Man and His Symbols*.

Superordinacy and Superordination

In contrast to Subordinacy, Superordination is a term used in logic to cover 'the Relation between a universal proposition and an individual proposition' (See any English Dictionary). And, immediately, we see that this relation is of tremendous importance because it ties in Logic to just about everything. This is not surprising in a world containing (supposedly) only relationships.

The list of applications is too long to furnish here, but I have in mind ideal forms, archetypes, specifications, embodiment, and so on, under the aegis of subjective probability linked with Information Theory. The essential features are that (a) there is a chain of Command or Authority and that (b) the levels in the chain are Relational.

For example, Jung's Trickster archetype should be 'Trickster and Victim', a generic Archetypal Form that could be played out (enacted) countless times in marginally differing ways each time. Similarly, each element of the *natural quaternion* is part of a relation that can be played out as a 'story' endlessly

SUPERCOMPUTERS

SUPERCONSCIOUS

William James

J.B. Priestley

SUPERVISOR (see Operating System)

SYSTEMS THEORY

General

Systems theory is not yet formalized as a coherent system of thought. It is, rather, a collection of individual 'system approaches', which are to some extent personalized but which come under that broad heading because they have attributes and functions in common. I usually work with reference to either Ludwig von Bertalanffy or Richard Mattessich (preferring the former to the latter).

Ludwig von Bertalanffy describes the different kinds of information that are available (their number is growing by the day). There is, at present, information qualified under 'cognitive', 'emotional', 'social', 'situational', 'environmental', 'political', 'classified', etc., all of which require the qualifications of context, theme, and appropriate priority value.

He points out that the most important factor in many judgments is that of *correct categorization*, and I have pointed out an example from personal construct theory in which wrong classification could have incurred an incorrect diagnosis. Dr. von Bertalanffy makes similar points in relation to systems balances and imbalances – and these apply to both living systems and non-living systems, i.e. Artificial systems.

Richard Mattessich complements these constructs by a treatise on *Instrumental Reasoning and Systems Methodology*, but over the use of this I urge a degree of caution. Whereas von Bertalanffy writes as a well-established biologist in relation to biological systems, Mattessich offers us a view that seems equally didactic and pompous but offers *ontological assumptions* and *unduly severe* criticisms of both von Bertalanffy and General System Theory, in general.

In particular, I urge caution because Mattessich, in my field of expertise, offers us opinions that are strangely lacking in 'contemporaneous modernity' at the time of writing. His book, *Instrumental Reasoning and Systems Methodology*, was published in 1978 and he cites L.J. Savage on Subjective Probability (pp.189-190) and completely ignores Jack Good, whose 'landmark in statistics' was published well before that year.

Mattessich's comments, in my opinion, suffer in quality as a consequence his limited references as well as the general loss of information affecting others. For example, he makes no mention of I.J. Good's 'landmark in the history of Statistics' (1950) cited as such by Savage in 1962 (with Barnard and Cox). [There is no mention in his Bibliography, either, of Barnard and Cox – and he *could* have mentioned my own linking of Subjective Probability with Information Theory in 1967 (!?)]

Applications

Mattessich's failings are probably more obvious to somebody actually working in the field of Real-Time Military Computer Systems, and my criticism does not matter particularly to many people. They are, however, real and they are significant. [This may reflect a difference between Academia and 'Workers in the Field']

He *does* provide us with useful information and opinions. I have in mind ideas such as *holistic dualism* and his five *Systems Principle*s of Polarity, Periodicity, Concrescence, Formative Preference, and Information. I therefore use him mainly as a source-book – rather than, say, for system design.

Additionally, to do him justice, Mattessich *does* indicate fleetingly an important branch of Analysis, called 'epitheoretical analysis', which includes 'a reconstruction of the background knowledge of social theories' and takes into account modal aspects – particularly normative and deontic factors. The 'social Leviathan', from von Bertalanffy, emphasizes the notion and its usefulness – albeit at Mattessich's cost.

Finally, I think it strange that Mattessich gives no mention of Relationism in a world consisting only of Relations and Fields (Smolin), and of computers thumbing, with gay abandon and with incredible speed, through relational and associative memories. His arguments, to me, seem very weak on the biological side of information-processing such as heuristics.

TAXONOMY OF SYSTEM TYPES

If we were to construct a complete taxonomy of system types, then – running through the levels – we would proceed through the descriptor-pairs (dichotomies), such as 'Physical / Transcendental' and 'Material / Non-Material', until we reached the level of 'Kingdom', which fortuitously has already been defined.

Therefore, at the categorical level of Kingdom, we could look specifically at 'Information – Processing' as a sub-kingdom and then identify 'Living' and 'Non – Living' as phyla. But, we would find a need for another phylum, that of 'Indeterminate' (which would contain within it a sub-category of 'Changeable'. After which, at the next level down , that of 'class', we would encounter some complexity because the descriptors 'Hybrid' and 'Indeterminate' re-appear.

The term, in fact, is applicable at every level – just as in Statistics the term 'something else' should always be included in the outlining of possibilities (even though it might have little likelihood of obtaining). Be that as it may, at a lower level still, say that of 'family' or of 'genus', we would discover that 'real intelligence is virtually indistinguishable from 'artificial' intelligence'. This relates to the animal kingdom only, because plants may be regarded as automatons by some.

This introduces another category in which fresh questions arise – about purpose, utility, volition, and so on. Plants are 'living bundles of conditioned responses' – they respond to stimuli in completely predictable ways. Apart from their qualities of Life they are as automatic as a clock. Or, so they would seem. If they *do* have *any* other qualities, such as feelings or the ability to be 'other than they are', then the living world is even more horrible than we can imagine.

It seems that we can rule out Intelligence as Nature's Aim. Perhaps Sherrington and Livesey (and others) are correct. It may well be that Emotion is equally important, but does that mean that elephants, whales, etc., can do what man has already done? What *is* the purpose behind Evolution? Suppose we look to Plato (again).

In this respect we can list his precepts – not necessarily in order of importance. First, draw no conclusions until we can explain the finest piece of matter. Second, control of one's self. Three, seek the Good and avoid the Bad. Fourth, seek 'Togetherness'.

Believe that seeking the Bad leads to metempsychosis. Sixth, work on the principle that only a philosopher of a lover with some knowledge of philosophy can reach 'transcendental re-union'.

If we are fully aware of Whitehead's remark that the history of philosophy is a series of footnotes to Plato, then we would not dream of 'challenging' him. But, Jung updated him, as Mons points out, and the updating can be improved by introducing the operations of *personal love* which Jung eschewed.

All that seems necessary is therefore to adjust Plato's sixth precept in terms of balance. This has to be done, in any case, if a Jung - Plato paradigm is to be established. A simple suggestion would be that we adjust the primacy and make Love equal in status to Intelligence or, perhaps better, Noesis, or Integrity, or Probity, or whatever.

This is in line with John Polkinghorne's adjustment of giving Plato's world equal stus to the material world – a very significant change in primacy. John Polkinghorne is an Anglican cleric as well as a Fellow of the Royal Society, and as such he believes in 'panentheism'. In other words the physical world is part of God but not the whole of God.

From our point of view it does not matter who or what is holding the universe together moment-by-moment. But, under Natural Theology, we can include the hypothesis within our considerations. Also, it is notable that Polkinghorne's high esteem for mathematical Platonism is consonant with that of Roger Penrose. Both sets of ideas converging, one might say, upon Donald MacKay's 'mechanistic embodiment'.

Indeed, contemplation of Taxonomy is likely, it seems, to emphasize and illuminate the mechanical nature of Existence. See Comprehensive Realism; Common Sense; Sex and Love; etc. However, within those fields we still have to account for the originator of the Command fiat *or* dispel the necessity for it (which can be done) See Pilot.

Returning to the issue of Taxonomy, the choosing of descriptors and levels is not only personal (to some extent) but is open to change as new information becomes available. For example, if we select – according to popular usage – a top level of 'Kingdom' (of Plants, Animals, Indeterminate), then it is only half-a-dozen levels of descent before we arrive at 'strain', whereat differences are comparatively slight.

The category of system labelled 'Information Processing' would be at a high level in the table because all living systems, it can be argued, process information in one way or another. And, we must bear in mind that Life cannot, yet, be adequately defined.

Thus we would sort through a variety of descriptors from which – according to our objective and perspective – we would attempt the task. Descriptors which come to mind, for example, are not easy to order in relation to each other when the terms 'User' and 'Used' are under consideration.

TEILHARD DE CHARDIN

For Teilhard the greatness of woman is less in her physical maternity (important and beautiful though this is) than in her spiritual fecundity; and the man-woman relationship, particularly in its celibate form, unleashes the greatest energy in the universe. This is the force that carries forward the thrust of life towards Omega, the personal centre of attraction, the ultimate point of convergence, the magnetic source of love from which nothing can separate us. In the final stage of unification in Omega, men will neither marry nor be given in marriage, 'but are like angels in heaven' (Mark: 12:25).

I include William Johnston's (above)citation (1976, pp. 157-8) of the Teilhardian conception of Omega, which is now largely rejected; but I neither accept it nor reject it, because I believe it to be fruitful. It pertains to a number of other features which I *do* accept. For example, it relates to the realm of the Superconscious, the Animus/Anima, the sense of Mission, Process Philosophy, Hinduism, Yin-Yang, Mysticism, Hidden Dimensions, and 'Elective Affinities' (of the kind that so fascinated Jung.

My reference to Elective Affinities leads naturally on to Plato's notion of 'part-souls' seeking re-unification, and these, perhaps, should be called 'Eclectic Affinities'. It leads, also, to an important philosophical difference between emergence and teleology (speaking loosely). Within Jung's ideology, being drawn to certain types is a straightforward feature of the accumulation of usable/discardable trivia.

With Plato, however, we have two *real* entities seeking each other out; and this is the main reason why I think Teilhard's theory was flawed. It is, in fact, to be expected that, *in hidden dimensions*, some higher form of consciousness should evolve - Superconsciousness – but I believe it is altogether too much to ask that a *soul* should evolve from a small piece of mind..

In a sense, therefore, the Omega concept does link a considerable number of significant phenomena together, and they all carry a substantial weight of evidence. The Superconscious, for example, has been posited from two different quarters in relation to medicine and the relationship between physical health and mental health. One source is cited by J.B. Priestley, in *Man and Time*, and the other is the report on *The Peckham Experiment* presented by Williamson and Pearse in *Science, Synthesis, and Sanity*.

THE WAY

Learning about Jung's ideology is like going to a wonderful production of an opera in which all the singers are excellent but one is very, very slightly unable to reach perfection. She engenders exasperation and pity in equal measure because she takes a fraction of a second to hit a high note or is just a shade off perfect pitch. The Jung-Plato Paradigm gives her both those qualities and makes her a diva.

Jung engenders exasperation because he is so manifestly inconsistent. Saying that he has experienced Love (p. 325) he abjures all 'emotional ties'. Referring to 'paradoxes' arising from Love, he asserts that no language is adequate to describe them. I wonder if he had read The Rubaiat or some of the Sufi works of Love. Modern poets are just as good.

Indeed, it has been argued for several hundred years that *only* poetry can convey the emotion. Within that field, Wordsworth is compared with Pope, and the Appendix contains a small selection which I have permission to print. But, the matter is wider and deeper than this. It extends into metaphors and into Perceived Ways of Life.

For example, Jung and Jungians categorize wrongly – and this is a cardinal sin (see von Bertalanffy). A fine example is that Odysseus is categorized as a Hero, when really that is a sub-category. In a world filled only with relationships, the proper main category is that of, say, 'Re-union'. Penelope plays her part – equally and admirably with Odysseus.

Likewise, the Trickster has Victims, and the Mother (by definition) has Offspring. In fact, all such talk can be categorized under two headings that reflect philosophical attitudes that are polar opposites of each other, namely Individualism and Relationism. Jung, for whatever reasons follow the former, whereas in Nature the latter obtains.

Jungians are fully aware of this – they call it the Jungian 'problematic' – and invariably they choose the direction 'Self' rather than 'Other'. And, this is a matter that stretches right back to the teachings of Gurdjieff who professed to know 'The Way'. His follower, P.D. Ouspensky, knew better and indicated the proper way through *Tertium Organum*.

TORUS

The mathematician, poet, and historian, Jacob Bronowski, remarked (BBC, Ascent of Man, 1973) that all living creatures are 'doughnuts – either solid or ring'. The quotation is memorable as an illustration of mathematical forms that can be approximated to any required degree of precision but never completely. This is because their respective mathematical formulae contain a 'transcendental' number, pi.

It follows that should either of their formulae be incorporated in a 'mechanistic embodiment' (as envisaged by Donald MacKay), then the embodied entity would also be transcendental. In the words of Rudy Rucker, a human being would be 'infinite-dimensional'. This would not have worried MacKay, because for him the ideal form lies embedded in the 'mind of God'. It shows to others, however, that the perfect ideal form of a human is likely to be *composite*.

Such a proposition is consonant with the notions of embodiment held by Jung, Plato, Hindus, and, in fact, with all who believe in some form of transcendental divinity. For Donald MacKay, it signifies a likelihood that the perfect ideal form needs to be approximated in the physical universe. In which case, Buddhism can be included in the set.

It also adds weight to the idea of Sherrington's imagined 'ultimate pontifical nerve-cell' – i. e. a 'Command element' – lying in the so-called 'psychical realm' as an individual but being elsewhere being part of a higher bipolar composite whole (see Motoyama).

Much of Roger Penrose's work is relevant to these matters (see, also, *Subjective Probability*), such as *ethereality*, *twistor theory*, and many mathematical notions pertaining to manifolds, patches, loops, dimensions, the human brain and protozoans, non-locality, and so on. Of particular interest, also, is the process of *transfinite induction* (see Daintith and Rennie, p. 221), and the Mandelbrot set (Penrose; Rucker). Both works emphasize the importance of *complex numbers*.

TRIUNE BRAIN AND TRIAGE BRAIN/MIND(EGO)

TRUTH

Plato made our decision making (Praxeology) easier for us by differentiating between two *categories* - 'Good' and 'Bad'. If we chose wisely (i.e. correctly) we would not only re-unite with the other part of our soul but we would also join (re-join) with God. He had in mind *Action,* and to this end he conceived of the simile of the *Charioteer*. For Plato, the Good is a generic terms covering Truth and Beauty and, presumably, their derivatives (in certain contexts and relating to particular themes).

Jesus Christ, some five hundred years later, proclaimed 'I am the Truth', and for him that meant agony on the cross in *self-sacrifice* for others. Pontius Pilate, contemporaneously, asked 'What is Truth?'. Both Jesus Christ and Pontius Pilate were speaking the truth from their different perspectives.

Nearly two thousand years later, 'Truth' was proclaimed as the 'first casualty of War. And, as I write, the term 'war' is being waged against religious fanatics, the various limbs of von Bertalanffy's 'social Leviathan', and arguably, accepting that Evil is determinant reality, the 'Principals' and/or 'Principles' of Evil, such as Satan and the conflicting efforts of minor gods.

Coming down to earth, with evolution, every 'living' entity (subject to definition) has needs which are governed individually by qualifiers of context and theme. There seems to be no exceptions to this observation – animals along the course of evolution (the 'living stream') are known to sacrifice themselves for 'others'. C.S. Sherrington made the point that 'Nature's Aim' seems to be that of developing 'Altruism as Passion'.

We can differentiate between *Truth, Honesty, Candour,* and *Falsehood*. The quartet form a *quaterninion* in the Jungian sense because there are four elements of *Quality* in the presentation of Information, of which one (Truth) is radically different from the others. This can be appreciated from the following loose definitions.

Truth

Truth is that which obtains in the absence of noetic manipulation and it is dependent upon the identification of context(s) pertaining to individual themes. It follows that Truth relates to the determination of the terms 'noesis', 'context' and theme, but this is not a barrier between human intelligence and artificial intelligence (see Penrose; Rucker; et al.)

Honesty is dependent upon noesis, and requires a noetic entity endeavouring to formulate truth without manipulating facts.

Candour differs from honesty in that it pays less heed to the feelings of others. It varies with cultures and it is dependent upon contexts re themes. (see von Bertalanffy)

Falsehoods involve intentionality. They can be benevolent or malevolent. They often involve relationships with others

From these loose definitions, we can conjecture that machine processing is the best way, in principle, of obtaining Truth. The snag arising in this conjecture is that programs have to be written by humans or by Dame Nature by way of genetics and the natural quaternion. Can such mechanisms avoid noesis? Can computer evolution 'breed out' noesis?

Subjective probability involves the assignment of numerical 'plausibility' to a *proposition* expressed in natural language, e.g. Is it going to rain soon? And, the proposition relates to a set of weighted indicators of likelihood, e.g. presence of certain types of cloud, prevailing winds, etc. if these can be coded, then the program can arrive at a conclusion on its own. Except that it has to be fed data about clouds, winds, etc., and *their* weightings as to those individual factors, by noetic entities. Or do they?

In short, can we ever, produce a computer system capable of making its own – completely impersonal – value judgments. One feels that such a computer system could only do so by heuristic methods. Even then, what would be the criteria of success? According to to Sherrington, Dame Nature's criterion is the quality of 'Altruism as Passion'.

And, within the constraints of Natural Theology, we can converge down to this concept but no further. Beyond this point we begin to perceive different 'perspectives' on that theme from the likes of May ('ontological necessity'), Ethel Person (Love as an 'Agent of Change'), Plato ('Re-union'), Whitehead ('Togetherness'), Johnston ('Merger' and 'Indwelling'), and, of course, a plurality of Poets.

Unless, that is, we conjecture that the very smallest entity possible is an element of *Experience*, and is a pole of a relationship, of which both poles have *Purpose*. This purpose – the subjective aim – is for concrescence. The system of thought producing these features is Whitehead's *Process Philosophy* – and who would argue against both Plato *and* Whitehead?

The question is rhetorical, because John Polkinghorne dares to amend Plato and to reject Whitehead. And, he is well qualified to do so – being both a Christian priest and a Fellow of the Royal Society. Polkinghorne, unfortunately, introduces an element of Faith into his arguments, but his words offer a platform from which to conduct our own investigations.

An example of this is his reference (1988, p. 57) to genetic mutations being a 'bias implanted in matter' (similar to Whitehead's 'subjective aim'). Polkinghorne says (correctly) that another way to describe this bias is to call it 'the Holy Spirit'. On the preceding page, he asserts (dubiously) that one reason for some scientists to incline towards the 'fanciful' idea of a demiurge at work is that they are unwilling to take account of religious experience.

Religious experience, he says, would point them to the *knowledge* (my italics) of a God transcendentally other and yet the ground of cosmic process. There is no mention of Hinduism, or the Sino-Asiatic model (described by Motoyama and by Jungian Timothy O'Neill) which offers almost exactly that.

John Polkinghorne criticises Paul Davies, Fred hoyle and others who espouse the 'demiurge model', yet the Christian apologist C.S. Lewis is willing to do. He re-iterates the Christian belief that the cosmos is not self-sustaining but is kept in being by a continuous act of will by its creator (p. 54)

Making the metaphysical assertion that the act of creation is a continuing process, he states that 'We reject the deistic idea that God simply lit the blue touch paper to set off the big-bang and then left the world to its own devices'. But this gives the wrong impression, Natural Theology affords us the avenue of prayer which may or may not be answered.

In this respect, Natural Theology, as presented by Alister Hardy, and Comprehensive Reality, as described by the late Donald MacKay, have a number of things in common. First and foremost may be that each has a deity responding to prayer. The former, Alister Hardy, introduces the notion of a change of direction analogous to the proper railway track to select, and the latter, Donald MacKay, provides for a state of grace to be obtained through a change in one's 'core of self-organization'.

Another cogent analogy is that the individual in both ideologies may be interpreted as moving along a 'story' that has already been written. We have the same interpretation as the one given by Omar Khayyam to the 'Moving Finger' that writes and having writ moves on. In mathematical Platonism, we have a 'wave of excitation' following choices of existing paths. The MacKay model affords little choice – other than to be different.

It is noteworthy that John Polkinghorne cites the concepts of set theory as being 'basic to all mathematics' (p. 75). And, he quotes the mathematician and logician Kurt Godel:

'Despite their remoteness from sense experience, we do have something like a perception of the objects of set theory, as seen from the fact that the axioms force themselves upon us as being true. I don't see any reason why we should have any less confidence in this kind of perception, i.e. mathematical intuition, than in sense perception'.

John Polkinghorne devoted more than a quarter of his book to Natural Theology, and a substantial part of this is addressed to quantum mechanics. However, mathematical Platonism avoids much of this – yet it does not dispute the reality of quarks and leptons. (see also Programs and Stories; Platonic World; Engine Driver; Bennett's Mathematical Model; etc.

TWISTOR THEORY

An approach to quantum gravity invented by Roger Penrose in which the primary elements are causal processe and the events of spacetime are constructed in terms of the relationships between the causal process (Smolin, p.220). The term 'causal processes' remind one of the 'causal plane' which makes sense in both Particle Physics and Hinduism.

The term 'processes', likewise, reminds one of Process Philosophy, Computer Systems, Ideal Forms, Embodiment, Time, and other relevant topics. In mathematics, 'twistors' are abstract geometrical objects which operate in a higher-dimensional complex space that underlies space-time (Martin Gardner, from Penroe, 1990, p. xv) See also Computers, Minds,

On page 483, Roger Penrose implies a metaphysical assertion that brain is a magnificent structure that *controls* our actions and somehow evokes an awareness of the world around (my italics). He then goes on to discuss 'Real Brains and Model Brains (pp. 483-522) and to ask the question 'Where lies the Physics of Mind?' (pp. 523-582).

Penrose remarks that 'beneath all this technicality is the feeling that it is indeed "obvious" that the *conscious* (his italics) mind cannot work like a computer, even though much of what is actually involved in mental activity might do so'. Our reasons may differ, but my own thesis is absolutely consonant with this – even though I endorse, almost completely, Donald MacKay's concept of Comprehensive Reality.

In this respect, twistor theory (Penrose), mechanistic embodiment (MacKay), Hinduism (Motoyama), and natural theology, all square with each other. Donald MacKay writes of divine acts of grace reaching into the core of our self-organization, and this is consonant with Alister Hardy's concept of divine response to prayer or in existential emergencies. Notably, twistor theory presents a non-local picture of space-time that involves complex numbers (Penrose, 1995, p. 389). See also *Ideal Forms.*

WARSHIP ANALOGY

Plato likened the psyche to the pilot of a ship. That vessel serves the Pilot, who at the time might have been regarded as a war leader. The modern warship – through its *real-time computer system* – serves its Command element in much the same way. Little is left for the Command element to do, other than to select a preferred action and to tell the system to engage in the activity, or not to do so, or to wait, in obeisance, for committal to one of the alternatives.

Popper and Eccles think that the simile is admirable and excellent (pp. 105-8; 120; 167, etc.), and Sherrington sees the human environment as 'akin to a battlefield, almost from end to end' (p. 293). MacKay models the workings of brain by the 'mind-like processes' of the 'Command support system', which is known today as an Intelligent Support System or 'ISS', and I add psychology to the MacKay model (see Comprehensive Reality).

All such viewpoints beg questions about the *User* of the ISS. Sherrington, although conceiving of brain collaborating with psyche, nevertheless suggests an ultimate pontifical nerve-cell with the brain and psyche being united in one entity. MacKay posits the mechanistic embodiment of an entity as a formula, communicating only with God. {see TORUS}

Popper and Eccles make an excellent case for the brain to operate in that fashion, but fail to give it any identity or autonomy. Ernest Kent runs completely parallel in his ideas (in that respect) but argues for monism. He thereby comes close to the mechanisms of the above authors, but fails to provide a satisfactory User.

WORLD-LINE

In Philosophy, a world-line is a line on paper representing an entity's passage through space-time – clearly there are missing dimensions. The power (usefulness) of a *torus* in mathematics is considerable. And organisms are 'doughnuts' – either ring or solid doughnuts (according to Bronovshi). It seems eminently reasonable, therefore, to conceive of a 'world line' being like a garden hose or a worm, and the world being the 'wormery' .

Some may prefer to use the latter simile because of the mating practice of earthworms. They 'couple' together by means of a shared surface area of 'interfacing' [not a lot of people know that]; and, this topological structuring might be called 'cohomology' or *holomorphic sheaf* cohomology by a mathematically inclined gardener or, better, a gardening mathematician. Roger Penrose calls the subject matter 'fairly sophisticated mathematical ideas' [whereupon I declare 'I pass'].

The salient point, for my thesis, is that the understanding of this correspondence between biology and mathematics promotes support for, and understanding of, not only Donald MacKays mechanistic embodiment but also the ease with which information processing and communication systems can merge.

We are taken very much deeper into mathematics by Roger Penrose in respect of his *Twistor Sheaf Cohomology* and his introduction of *infinitesimals* (2004, p. 987), which relate to Realms further along the Axis of Scale (such as the Hindu levels of divinity outside the physical universe.

YIN-YANG

The YIN and the YANG, respectively, are long-held by many to be principles of *femininity* and of *masculinity* that co-operate with each other in the LIFE FORCE driving a 'spiritual' entity. I take the term 'spiritual' to mean 'within the physical universe' and not to mean 'transcendental', which is outside the physical universe. I make this point because there is confusion about the status of 'spirit' and 'soul'.

In the Asiatic and Oriental countries – especially the whole stream of Sino-Japanese culture and Hinduism – Yin and Yang are contained within the spiritual entity when it is *outside* the physical universe: they are released when the spiritual entity is *inside* the physical universe so as to drive or to *manifest as*, respectively, women and men. (YIN precedes YANG in the Asian and Eastern regions as an indicator of their equality).

Jung posited a LIFE FORCE and, similarly, he distinguished between EROS and LOGOS. He and his disciples failed, however, to furnish the age-old symbol of equality. In *Man and his Symbols* they relied on the I CHING and *soothsaying* in clinical practice rather than the more appropriate Yin-Yang; and Jung played down the importance of personal love, but gave one (long) paragraph on *cosmogonic* love.

The concept of Yin and Yang being, respectively, female and male principles, has been built up over five thousand years by disciplined thought and acute observation coupled with controlled imagination.   Today it is represented mathematically by corresponding sets of odd/even numbers representing the difference in effect throughout Nature.

In fact, today we can do better than this. We can represent them in more detailed set theory and actually model their conjectured co-operation within one spiritual body – as it is perceived conjecturally (with some supporting evidence).

Initially, the two individual series of even and odd integers can be arranged into one series of ordered pairs. As Yin and Yang are expressed deliberately in that order to indicate absolute equality (a point overlooked by Jung) there is no necessary preference for one gender over the other, but M and F can in any case be changed to equal poles and opposite directions, such as N(orth) and S(outh).

The two principles, at work, can then be interpreted as Northerly and Southerly winds blowing alternately upon clothes along a washing line resulting in an ever-changing topological material structure – especially if we make the weather conditions very changeable. And, this notion comes close to considerations in mathematical physics of *symmetry* and, for want of a better word, *propinquity*.

This points up the dire error in Jung's avoidance of human sexual relationships, and has practical significance when it is found that *all* of the characteristics of Personality that Jung attributed to a hypothesized psychic system – separate and distinct from the material body – are, indeed, attributable to an inert, real-time, intelligent, *computer system*.

It is singularly strange that Jung posited a *Life Force* and two principles, the *Logos* and Eros, perceivable in the Sino-Asiatic model, but failed to incorporate them into his private life or his public pronouncements.   [He had, of course, painted himself into a corner by his private affairs]   And so it remained until Timothy O'Neill rectified the error by allegory and the works of Donald MacKay on mechanistic embodiment established O'Neill's allegory by the provision of computer models.

This is accentuated by the fact that Jung had other knowledge available to him that he seems either to have neglected or ignored. I refer to the *Natural Quaternion* which is formed of four elements which are *Relationships*, of which one is clearly different from the others. Namely, this is the set of : Parent, Offspring, Sibling, Other.

The accentuation is reinforced by the acceptance of many modern Jungians that the Other is part of their 'problematic'. It will remain so until they accept the evidence I produce of the conclusive isomorphism between the human 'Brain/Mind(Ego)' and a special-purpose real-time computer system (see Taxonomy)

There is more to this, however, because the locating of Personality in the Brain/Mind(Ego), i.e. what might be called 'biological personality', is virtually 'evolutionary personality'. It can be traced back to Roger Penrose's *paramecium* and to my *chlamydonas*, i.e. to unicellular creatures and effects upon them *from their environments.*

Roger Penrose argues that, paired cells are 'non-local' and are joined or linked by properties of the cell structure, other than the nucleus. He identifies the *cilia* as the agents of this. And, Timothy O'Neill's version of Jungian theory indicates that *Yin* and *Yang* (in the guise of *Anima* and *Animus*) reflects correctly the separating out of Yin and Yang from the 'spirit-body' in the physical universe. It is noteworthy that, apparently, the 'pairing' involved in both representations comes from the same non-local mechanism.

In addition, my earlier, and loose, chain of events from set theory to Yin/Yang may well involve something like, conjecturally, a 'solenoid'. And, indeed, the organization of nucleosomes and spacer regions of a cell do involve the 'solenoid model' in which 6-7 nucleosomes are grouped together at a time, *and* branches of *beating cilia* (in humans) propagate currents of a liquid.

So now there are two or three putative arguments for outside physical effects upon individual cells. It does not follow that the source of such input is transcendental (in the normal course of events) and it is adequately accounted for by the action of Yin and Yang upon the material entities from the *causal plane* through the *upper and lower astral planes* as *in* the normal course of events.

ZOHARIAN INTERFACE

The subject-matter of Danah Zohar's very useful book, *The Quantum Self*, is similar to the book written separately and independently by David Hodgson, an Australian high court judge. On page seven of his book, *The Mind Matters*, Hodgson expresses his belief about Science in the Modern World.

His belief is that science in the 20th. Century, if properly understood, is consistent with, and supports, the view that reality is not essentially material. This belief , also, is that consciousness is important and causally relevant, and that values are not merely subjective or illusory. Hodgson tries to make good these beliefs in reference to topics such as computers, causation, reasoning, and evolution.

On reading a book for the first time, it is surprisingly useful to take a summary prior look at its name index and subject index. Hodgson's indexes do not disappoint. The 'usual suspects' are included and the works of Plato, Aristotle, Ouspensky, Whitehead, Cantor, May, and others, are absent.

However, Philosophy is mentioned on Page eleven and (looking on the bright side) Hodgson *does* refer to Hofstadter's prize-winning book, *Godel, Escher, Bach*, in favourable terms.

That book, says Hodgson, is persuasive in its suggestions of how intelligent and purposive behaviour can be exhibited by the interactions of non-intelligent and non-purposive units. Without further ado, therefore, readers are reminded that the kind of real-time computers dealt with by Donald MacKay are composed of the most-basic material elements and have intelligence in some ways superior to humans, and they share the same features of Personality, but they exist to serve a User of a *different kind*.

Bearing this in mind, a return to John Polkinghorne's diatribe on the Demiurgoi indicates that his book, *Science and Creation,* in Shakespeare's words 'protests too much' about the matter. Indeed, the work is so filled with many contradictions and paradoxes that it is *almost* useless for any epitheoretical purpose.

Indeed, it can be surmised that a majority of epitheoretical analysts and observers would support many of the propositions that John Polkinghorne rejects. [One criticizes the argument but certainly not the man] And, they might well centre upon Danah Zohar's pantheistic approach to quantum theory. Especially as Dr. Polkinghorne's other book, *The Quantum Universe*, is less burdensome in such respects.

The book, however, *does* take quantum uncertainty as a metaphysical assertion, without considering alternatives – Roger Penrose shows how this should be done, and in fact he espouses the same cause – of mathematical Platonism – as is taken in this monograph.

This does not mean that its underlying religious theme is pantheistic – except, perhaps, in the way that the Hindu yogic traditions views Existence asa hierarchy of spirit bodies including levels of divinity and the physical universe. This flatly contradicts the assertion of John Polkinghorne of equality of status between the material and the spiritual (which he calls 'mental', page 77).

Danah Zohar's concept of 'wave-particle duality' involves an interface which savours of Command input to the material brain, and the radical flaw in her philosophy can be represented in a single sentence, or proposition, on page 158 of *The Quantum Self* with regard to this feature.

Danah Zohar states

'It is only with a quantum model of the person, where "I-ness" arises out of a coherent, unifying quantum state in the brain, that there can be any one central "me" who makes or avoids mistakes' (p. 158)

This proposition arises from a supposition which states, immediately before her statement, that 'I-ness' inevitably fragments otherwise into 'a tangled mess of individual neurones'; and this is not so.

Before explaining how the 'tangled mess' of neurons is, in fact, a highly organized, hierarchical, tiered , material system producing 'I-ness', we can consider the Zoharian interface, per se.   The model of this, so to speak, is of a 'ghostly' hand of bosons playing upon an appropriate instrument (say, q piano),

Perhaps, a more accurate metaphor would be *two* ghostly hands setting the beads of an abacus spinning in either of two directions, but that (pardon the pun) is immaterial. Danah Zohar posits that the 'body' to which the hand belongs is formed, one might say, by the 'tangled mess' of waves emanating from a mass of relationships (in the material world).

In fact, the fact of particle physics, the shifting and shaping of the 'hand' is conducted through leptons and quarks at a lower level (not mentioned by Danah Zohar). And, it is at *this level* that the Yin and Yang principles operate (freely) in the physical universe to give femaleness and maleness.

Jung calls them by a different name, with slightly differing properties, but they are essentially the same within the Life Force – except that Jung sees them as being contained always within a 'spirit body', but he is wrong on this, because, in the physical realms, Yin and Yang are liberated (see Motoyama).

[It must be said that the Zoharian explanation (at the bottom of page 158) of the mechanism of the Bose-Einstein in producing a correlated effect on the brain's neurons in *not* being challenged]

And so, returning to the Zoharian 'tangled mess of neurones', the best place to start is perhaps with the words of Sherrington and then to move on to computer models – in a completely appropriate way.   Sherrington depicted a brain organized under a 'principle of convergence' which converged upon, at the apex, an 'ultimate pontifical nerve-cell'.

His words are not always clear, but he postulated also that brain collaborates with psyche and, therefore, it seems open for us to speculate somewhat about the interface between brain and psyche.   Wherever we may choose to seek this interface it appears to promote the easiest possible decision-making, such as a simple, 'Yea', 'Nay', or 'Stay' concerning a course of action proffered by the brain.

This is eminently reasonable because Sherrington perceived that Man's environment is akin to a battlefield, far and wide. It is not surprising that a special purpose, real-time computer system should be used in a military role to defend and to nurture man's fellows.   This is *not* inany way connected with *self*-preservation. Quite the opposite obtains – the warship and its personnel are expendable, provided the *Mission* is completed.

All of this is consonant with the reduction of Jung's notion of a psyche by the encephalization of the 'mind(Ego)' and the close correspondence between the 'brain/mind(Ego) and the attributes and functions of a real-time military computer system.   The closeness is so great that Jung's complete concept of *'Personality'* accompanies the encephalization.

The analogy, i.e. the *isomorphism'*, is so cogent, also, that Donald MacKay's *Comprehensive Reality* pursues, in parallel, the theme of *mechanistic embodiment* in terms of *'the mechanization of mind-like processes'*.   MacKay conceives of the whole *organism* being an embodied mathematical formula, in which there are two functionaries.

The first such functionary is called the Agent, i.e. the real-time computer system, and the other is called the Determinator, echoing the Command function at its most simple – as indicated above.   And, in contrast to Danah Zohar proclamations to the contrary (p. 158), the Agent is perfectly capable of acting on its own initiative.

The term 'encephalization of the Mind(Ego)' is more specific – especially in regard of Jungian theory – than MacKay's 'mechanization of mind-like processes', but both terms refer to exactly the same kind of real-time computer system.   MacKay's replacement of a computer screen by a batch of arrays, memories, etc., etc., is not quite achievable yet, but we are very nearly 'there'.

Therefore, Ludwig von Bertalanffy's 'perspectivism' comes into play and various inter-linked topics can be understood and appreciated (and used) better by that viewpoint.   Readers are requested, consequently, to look at the following entries in the Glossary/Guide in the following (loose) order: Mission and Command, Moral Responsibility, 'I', Agents.

Bearing in mind the difficulties of translation, it is possible to discern one source of error in Jung's book, *Memories, Dreams, Reflections*, by going right down to his basic individual wording.   If we do this we find, at times, that Jung's ideas seem closer to Natural Theology than to Christianity.   But, having said this, one thinks immediately of his reference (p. 306) to the dogma pf the Catholic church.

It savours of nit-picking but it has to be done.   In a sense, this is a tribute to Jung because the need arises from the coherence and consistency and coherence of his ideas – it is the direction in which they point that needs correction.   A comparison (one of many possible comparisons) can be made with the MacKay model, i.e. an organism as an embodied formula.

We start with Jung's metaphysical assertion that 'at bottom' the psyche is simply 'world' (p. 357)   [The deeper 'Layers' of the psyche are universalized and extinguished in chemical substances].   This is completely in accordance with MacKay, Sherrington, Zohar, et alia., until we define chemical substances in terms of atoms composed of Fermions acted upon by Bosons.

Thereafter, we have to consider the Zoharian interface between Fermions and Bosons and the nature of those subatomic particles.   The difference between them is called a 'dualism of properties', and the system of bosons – which changes from moment-to-moment – we can call, for the sake of argument, a psyche (which is not transcendental but part of Jung's 'world' [i.e. Existence, or the physical universe, or the solar system]

At this (secondary) level there is no way in which Jung's concept of a psyche can obtain.   The next level (tertiary) level is the one in which leptons and quarks fashion fermions and bosons.   And, at this level, we start to encounter the hierarchy of 'spiritual bodies' described so well by Hiroshi Moyoyama in presenting the conceptual system that follows the Hindu yogic tradition.

Loosely speaking, this practical school of thought conceives of a spiritual body at all levels of Existence, each of which is powered by a Life Force and the co-operating principles of Yin and Yang. Inside the lowest level, i.e. the physical universe, the yin and yang are manifested *outside* the spiritual body so as to formulate (through the tertiary level) female and male organisms.

In the physical universe, therefore, the co-operation between the Yin and the Yang principles takes the form of bipolar relationships, which individually or as a pair, have tasks to complete successfully before the principles can re-engage with each other inside the spirit body, whereupon it can ascend to a higher (transcendental) level. Plato, and others, would have them seeking each other – this is an idea which captivates human beings.

Timothy O'Neill visualizes this 'affinitive search' notion to perfection in *The Individuated Hobbit*, and if we follow Plato, then the Jungian concept of Anima/Animus becomes completely understandable and acceptable to everybody. To everybody, that is, except Jung, who had painted himself into a corner in his private and personal life.

He seems to have been in a position, regarding his wife, mistress, and a number of other ladies, in which he could not possibly identify such an entity as a 'soul-mate'. Whatever his reasons, Jung chose to incorporate into his ideology an idea which, at best, can only be described as 'Fatuous'.

In this situation, Jung found his individualistic ideas threatened by the irresistible rising tide of *Relationism*. And so we are left – even today – with the incredible notion that the psyche, throughout aeons of experience, gathers up features of *real* women and builds them into *fictive* pictures of women that lead, eventually, to one final image of a fictive 'target' woman which can be used within the organism and then discarded.

If the above description is correct (and I have read, and re-read, the tract many scores of times), then it leads to all kinds of threats from inside and outside the human organism; and it is not surprising that it is still called (see Papadopoulos) the Jungian 'problematic'. For the basis of Psychology and Psychiatry it is positively dangerous.

However, it no longer obtains, because (a) Timothy O'Neill has corrected it and (b) the whole thrust of Jung's fundamental concept of *Personality* has been switched from <u>*Self*</u> to <u>*Other*</u>. Those two factors brings the (corrected) Jungian theory fairly and squarely in line with the Hindu yogic tradition – having restored the damage done to it by Jung. They also bring it into consonance with Plato.

(See, also, Myths and Irrationality)

APPENDIX

This Appendix is a condensation of material which I had intended to cover three aspects of my personal life – (a) my visions and personifications akin to those of Jung, (b) my choice of the scientific revelations emanating from poetry, and (c) further examples from my published works.

I soon decided, however, that any further examples of my previous research would be quite superfluous to the main thrust of my argument – I had said enough. Following this, on looking back through discarded drafts, much the same seemed to apply to my selection from poetry, although three examples are so pertinent to the Jung-Plato paradigm that I include them.

Most of my visions and personifications are quite similar to Jung's (one of them included Jung) and have special features justifying their inclusion. There are several which are highly personal and which I exclude – they are those which feature some statistically significant pieces of information, and readers, I fear, will have to take my professional word on their significance.

One of the exclusions surprised me mightily. It was what Jung would have called an 'encounter with an archetype'; and, although I would like to have included it, I do not do so because it is too personal. I can say, however, that the experience lived up to his description of such an encounter, but I am reasonably sure that no part of my own organism could have produced such awe-inspiring power, intensity and presence.

I start, therefore, with three pieces of poetry which speak for themselves. The first is by Harold Pinter, and I have permission from his publishers (Methuen) to print it:-

I know the place

I know the place.

It is true.

Everything we do

Corrects the space

Between death and me

And you.

The second poem needs no permission to print because it is mine – under the *nom de plume* of Lance Cogar. It is even shorter than Pinter's.

<u>*Statement of Fact*</u>

I did,

Still do,

And always will

Love you.

My third selection is printed with permission from *The Mathematical Gazette*. It is by Ms. Ann M. Atkin, and this lady shows a very fine and pleasing touch. Her poem runs:

Somewhere,

At a place they call infinity,

Where centres of curvature of straight lines

Lurk around corners,

And pairs of parallel lines

Have orgies of touching one another,

The last figure of Pi

Sits in regal majesty

On the focus of a parabolic straight line,

And root two is feeling more rational than usual,

If you look hard enough

You can see the reciprocal of zero has just found its value,

A converging series has just lost its common ratio,

And two curves are looking to see if his B2 equals her 4AC,

And there on the floor is a note that says 'I love you'

From you to me.

From Anne Atkins' splendid poem it is but two short steps to Platonism. The first is a step backwards in Time by some four hundred years to the poetry of John Donne. This keeps us within the same context and theme, but effuses a somewhat deeper sense of Mysticism and Affinitive Search.

By this, I mean the concept of each incarnation as a person – in an affinitive relationship – being a _pole_ of an _Ideal Form_. The ideal form represents _exactness_, but the poles are (by Plato's definition) _inexact_. Following MacKay, we can think, then, in terms of 'embodied' mathematical formulae. This is Step Two, and it may one day lead us into 'Supersymmetry'.

As an example, we have that a certain famous scientist regarded people as sets of differential equations, but did not dare tell his wife of that view of her. Accordingly, the recollection of their wholeness together – seated in the 'core' of each pole's 'centres' of self-organization priority-evaluation (MacKay) - would be exact, but the results of the self-organization would be inexact (and much as Freud envisaged)..

It follows from this that, during a series of incarnations, each pole (of an affinitive pair) could encounter any number of approximate 'near misses' and probably a number of encounters with the 'real thing'.   The former might produce some instances of 'falling in love', so to speak, but the latter might well require learning and appreciation of the affinitive pole's qualities.   In short, it would be one of the forms of mystical love.

The _nuances_ of this seem to be most apposite in John Donne's poem, which includes the lines:-

'Twice or thrice had I loved thee

Before I knew thy face or name.

So in a voice, so in a shapeless flame,

Angels affect us oft, and worshipped be'.

Finally, I quote Richard Lovelace, whose sentence should be a watchword for every lover, bar none.

I could not love thee (Dear) so much,

Lov'd I not honour more.

To Lucasta, Going to the Wars.

Little further comment is needed, except that I believe the poem of Ann Atkins to be a very wonderful love-poem in which all kinds of relevance to my theme can be found.

The group of visions and personifications which follows, from my own experience, presents a very different 'kettle of fish' which _does_ seem, however, to reflect the inadequacy not only of our knowledge, but also the limitations of our thought processes. Except, that is, for the pairing of Jung's functions of Intuition and Feeling, backed by Ouspensky's _Tertium Organum_.

Everybody, for example, perceives a need for extra dimensions, some schools of thought actually posit them and work through them, but everybody wishes also, so to speak, paddle their own canoe. As Moriarty said to Holmes, 'It won't do' (or *vice-versa*).

Our inability to tie down extra-sensory perception is an example of this. Its irregularities offer backing for those professing a need for extra dimension coming from all quarters, and the 'road of the East' offers centres (chakras) and channels (nadis) through which energies may be marshalled and communicated.

We find, too, that extra dimensions are being posited for Space, Time, Scale, Knowledge, and Emotion. And all of this is apparently catered for in the Sino-Asiatic model. But, what about the claims by excellent scientists that there are only Relationships and Fields? Nearly all of the research carried out so far has been in regard of Individualism, which metaphorically speaking, is _dead_, having given way to _Relationism._

And so, it is against this background that I present my own (apparently) mystical experiences involving (apparently) Others. Clearly, much of the detail comes from my own mind, but equally each contains also some function, event, or detail of which I was completely unaware at the time (such as Jung's *penchant* for the music of brass bands). So, without further ado, I offer the following:-

Personification One

This single 'dream' took place over a continuing sequence of four 'scenes' – as in a film. Only one scene (the second) features Jung, but they are all part of the same 'story'. The theme of this story is my correction of his ideology despite his objections.

The background of the story is my change of heart over Jung (at the time) which had been increasing steadily over a score of years. I was becoming vexed by the string of inconsistencies, ambiguities, misconceptions, and other obfuscations in his writings caused by factors in his private life. These had been well-chronicled already, and I had no wish to refer to them.

The contents of each scene followed each other neatly in passing time – just as chapters in a work of fiction. Each was in colour and was filled with appropriate descriptive detail. Only the second scene contained intercommunication, but not in sound or sign.

Only the fourth scene contained sound, and this was of a brass band playing quite loudly against a subdued background of 'community' noise, such as children at play, grown-ups chatter, etc. At the time, I was unaware of Jung's liking of such music; and this 'dream' seemed so 'portentous' that I took pains to record these details immediately on waking up.

Scene One

This was of a dry, dusty, derelict and almost deserted landscape, similar to the 'dustbowl' or wasteland of the USA. It was of the kind that was particularly well-suited to the works of John Steinbeck. The feeling generated by the scene was so strong that on awakening I looked up T.S. Elliot's poem, The Wasteland, to confirm the impression and its *ambience*.

The scene was so strongly etched into my mind that, even now almost thirty years on, it comes readily to mind in almost every detail. The predominant colour was sandy-yellow, and it seemed to tinge even the pale-blue of the cloudless sky. The monotony of colour was relieved only by the patches of pale, faded brown provided by a few, scattered ramshackle shacks.

Several of these unappealing buildings had a dishevelled adult sitting on a veranda or on the steps leading to a veranda. A few ragged children played desultorily in the dust, and one or two lean dogs were foraging listlessly around. Silence reigned, as did a tremendous feeling of torpor and inertia. I was making my way through this landscape, unheeded and unheeding, but (so far as I can remember) I had no clear purpose in mind.

Scene Two

Suddenly, the scene changed completely. It was, however, in keeping with and continuous with the first scene, and I felt no disruption. I was now climbing up a rather narrow flight of steps – as in a cinema, theatre, or lecture hall - belonging to a typical (or so it seemed) 'small town' lecture theatre or town hall.

It was not large, and it was somewhat unkempt; and it had a tiered seating arrangement sweeping round in a semi-circle focused upon a small dais, with a lectern and a very ordinary blackboard and easel. The room barely warranted the title of 'hall' or 'theatre' but, nevertheless, those were the terms that entered my mind.

A small man in a black gown, and wearing a mortar-board, was writing on the blackboard and I knew it was Jung. He had rather less hair than I would have expected, and the figure was more slight and less impressive than the pictures of Jung that I had seen in books. However, the face was clearly recognisable.

As I recorded this phenomenon the following morning, I became further convinced of my impression by seeing that, written on the blackboard, there was nothing arcane or erudite but merely a cooking recipe, which I instantly associated with alchemy. On this, I started to move towards the doorway, whereupon he was instantaneously confronting me, blocking my exit. He had swelled up hugely – as 'genies' do on release from their captivity – and he looked *almost* threatening, but not quite so. [On reflection, I thought *forbidding* was more appropriate.]

No words were exchanged between us, but I divulged my thesis to him in one instantaneous burst of information transfer – I could almost hear it and feel it. At the time (the early 1980s), such transfers of very highly condensed sets of data were completely unknown to me (and were probably in their infancy) although I had done some rudimentary work on text-compression.

Upon receipt of this packet of densely compressed information (my thesis), the figure resumed its normal size and stood back to allow me to go past. He seemed almost reluctant to do so, but not quite. He was almost smiling, but not quite. I felt that my thesis and my credentials had been accepted, and went on my way.

Scene Three

Again there was an abrupt change of scene. This time I found myself in very familiar territory – I knew it very well indeed. Long ago, before ASWE was built, it had been a very narrow road, with tall hedgerows, which ran through farming country and led to a cross-roads before opening out. The road was well-known to me because, at that time, I had walked with a girlfriend(s).

Since then the road had widened – after ASWE had been built – but it was still narrow and hedged. Primarily, though, my familiarity with this stretch of road stemmed from my driving along it (twenty-five years later) four times a day for twenty-five years. And, this time there was a difference – a vast difference (in my dream).

The road beyond the crossroads had been blocked off. It was completely filled with rack upon rack of razor wire and barbed wire. A number of black, sinister, hooded lenses (similar to the head of a cobra) swooped, here and there, and peered at me, suspiciously and menacingly. They were mounted on telescopic necks, resembling swan necks, of light chain mail.

This brooding inquisitorial surveillance reminded me strongly of the Martian invaders from the film, *War of the Worlds*, after the Martians had landed. Presumably, these images had been taken from my mind's data banks to fashion the scene in which I found myself. Despite the appearance of suspicion and menace, I felt completely unperturbed and at ease.

Scene Four

It was obvious that the way ahead was utterly impenetrable – forbidden. And, upon this acceptance, I found myself in Scene Four. I was proceeding 'back', but along an entirely different route, and a different *kind* of route. Now, the scenery was vivid and intense. The roadway was smooth, broad and open.

It was bordered by sumptuous buildings and luscious, green parks and gardens. I could hear festive brass bands playing buoyant tunes; and I could just see the bands, with their uniformed and capped musicians, through the trees, which were in full foliage. There were crowds of lively, cheering, waving, adults intermingling with noisy, excited children. _Everything_ seemed easier, smoother, more festive, and altogether more welcoming.

Discussion

I must point out, immediately, that I was completely unemotional throughout all four scenes. I detest Triumphalism [and I can justify this claim]. I find it abhorrent partly because it does not seem to 'run' in any of my discernable forebears, and also because my schools, my military service, and my close friends, forbade it – it was not done. Thus, I _do_ find Scene Four difficult to explain – or, rather I _did_.

For a long time the analysis of this dream puzzled me – it seemed, for example, too long, too continuous, and too coherent for a dream. Scene Four smacked strongly of triumphalism, which was not in my nature or nurture. And I felt strongly that it was all in my 'n-dimensional' neural circuits.   Then, when the assembly of the Jung-Plato paradigm came to completion, it all became – almost instantly – clear and comprehensible.

I had been wrong in perceiving Scene Four as different and 'over-hyped'.   The whole personification 'story' had seemed exaggerated, because it was _allegorical_.   This meant that it was a communication – and an 'internal' or 'mental' one, to boot.   It was strictly in accordance with the paradigm, in which Donald MacKay's _Determinator_ represents the situation to his _Agent,_ or _vice-versa._

My second personification also involves apparent inter-communication between 'Self' and 'Other', but this time the whole incident smacks of reality.   In the manner of the relationship between Timothy O'Neill's 'Goldberry' and Tom 'Bombadil', I speae in natural language, and my 'psychagogue' (in the Jungian idiom) immediately plants information in my mind.   Neither do I remember actually hearing sound as I speak.

Personification Two

I was walking through the iron gates of a university with my psychagogue, who was completely swathed in white apart from her eyes in the Arabic mode..   As we walked across the quadrangle, I asked for her name.   Immediately, the name 'Rosamunda' entered my mind.   This held very vague recollections for me, so I checked with her – spelling out the name in two syllables, and giving it a very loose translation – something akin to 'rose of the world' or 'flower of the field'.   She nodded.

Then we entered a university lecture hall and climbed to the top of a precipitous stairway from which the dais seemed very distant.   This encounter lasted only a short time, and I took it to be an unambiguous signal from 'Rosamunda' to continue distancing myself from Academe.

This interpretation was in keeping with my experience.   For decades, I had felt a kind of 'guidance' over decisions that I had learned to trust [as did Jung], but this encounter was the only 'Self to Psychagogue' experience of which I am aware.   Apart from the experiences that I am withholding, I have experienced about half-a-dozen which are not so noteworthy as these two.

These other instances involved, variously, touch, sight (colour), communication, precognition (once), activity, and meaning, and they followed much the same patterns as has been claimed by authorities on mysticism.   However, following Priestley's opinion, I believe that they are far more commonplace than is recognised – as is the wealth of hypnagogic equipment in our brains available to our imaginations.

For me, Personifications One and Two forms a radical triage of corrections to Jungian theory that enables, or makes a gateway for, the raising of Jungian psychology to the level of Platonism.   The former shows that *Personality* is not only a feature of the evolutionary brain and its functions and attributes, but also (seemingly) a general characteristic of all 'real-time information processing systems'.

The latter substantiates two corrections that have a great impact.   First, it pairs Jung's function of Intuition with that of Feeling.   Second, it supports Timothy O'Neill's correction of Jung's misinterpretation of Hindu philosophy, which reaches down into therapeutic practice. In short, it makes the Anima/ Animus a _real_ entity.

This set or triage of amendments makes the Jung-Plato not only possible, but viable and desirable. _And_, it is in accordance with all the experience and wisdom of 'the road of the East' as it joins with 'the road of the West'.

Furthermore, it has an effect completely against the grain of my determination to be rigorous. It leads me to identify for readers a work by Michael Talbot, called _The holographic Universe_, which I had never, ever, thought of praising. I'd always held it in high regard as a source-book for 'p-baked' ideas, but among all the messy and sloppy (and dangerous) thinking it records, there is commentary on the place of holography in future science that ties-in neatly with 'twistors', spin-networks, symmetry, supersymmetry, Riemannian space, Hinduism, etc., etc.

In regard of mysticism within the physical universe, it just cries out for representation in an epitheoretic web of the kind I have shown in Part Three. Readers should, however, proceed with great care because Talbot's coverage does not include critical commentary, and some of his contributors ascribe to practices of the kind that have been made illegal in some places.

Finally, I feel that an explanation may be warranted concerning my occasional references to Jung being a victim of his nature, nurture and circumstances, while, in this Appendix particularly, I seem to share those of his experiences and opinions which I appear to decry.

For example, having (almost) completely dismissed myths as being survival mechanisms or instruments of war, or wishful thinking and persuasion, etc., why do I cite poems which seem to present truths? The answer to any question of that nature is that my own nurture, nature, and circumstances, _do_ (of course) affect my analysis and observations of daily life. Intakes of coffee and of alcohol come readily to mind as examples,

And, overall, my thoughts _are_ shaped towards mathematical Platonism and the Hindu yogic tradition, but such thoughts and movements are not appropriate to the attempted rigour of the monograph. I suppose it can be argued that, in reaching into Sapientia and its mystical processes, I am achieving a transcendence that is beyond Rigour and has become Knowledge.

Moreover, it can be argued that poetry is a form of information transfer that is separate and distinct from prose. Were this a treatise, rather than a monograph, I would quote substantially to this affect from the Folio Society's publication of _A Short History of English Literature_ by Gilbert Phelps. He dwells much on poetry as the revelation of Truth, and I have permission to quote as much as I wish. Much the same can be said about Music, a really powerful case can be made for the 'mechanization of musical processes'.

Following from this, it is but a short step for one who has _experienced_ the so-called stages of the growth of a fictive, stochastic and disposable Anima/Animus, to join with

Ruth Munroe and cry, 'Rubbish'. The same applies to archetypes. All the grouping and categorization of archetypes, in a world acknowledged to be Relational, should be relational.

As I write, it is about eighty-four years since I started to make action decisions based upon situation analysis. Since leaving school, I have felt increasingly that I am an 'Agent', following some prescribed coure and guided by an Overseer or 'Determinator'

All in all, therefore, a companion volume is being prepared which covers all these absent features. I think I will call it *The Life and Times of a Naval Scientist* and assure readers that it will completely *underexpurgated*. Life, in general, and Science, in particular, have been very 'good' to me, and it will give me great pleasure to share some of the laughter, tears, sport, and camaraderie that I have experienced and to reveal some of the wondrous depths of emotion that can be encountered in the search for Truth.

This having been said, such an autobiographical work will still need, I feel, some initial section explaining how Ouspensky's Intuitional Logic become entwined with Mathematical Platonism in the generation of Experience.

Returning to the present, in Part Three, I offer an 'n-dimensional' matrix or 'grid' which serves several purposes. First, it provides a Glossary for the contents of Parts One and Two. Second, it furnishes a kind of multi-dimensional 'road map' of the philosophical ground covered in general by Science in the modern world. Equally, it can be used by anyone with sufficient interest, because none of the categories and interconnections is fixed rigidly.

An interested layman, for example, could either use my 'Guide' as a starting point or could start from scratch on the construction of his/her own body of findings. In either case, their individual creations would provide a fertile ground for cross-comparisons with others. In principle, this could be done to good effect on a computer (provided that international agreement could be reached).

Because my own research findings overlap with numerous others I am forced to use the first person singular in Parts One and Two. My experience is intimately linked also with others, but in this case the opposite applies. I cannot be specific and so the material of Part Three is completely personal but not open to public scrutiny.

Part Three, therefore, tends to be more academic and didactic in its presentation. I'm afraid that this is unavoidable, and I can only apologise to readers. I hope readers will understand that this is, to some extent, a matter of mood.

To sum up, therefore, Jung's prescription of *Personality* to a supposed non-material has defects which lead to serious repercussions in other parts of his work. For example, they affect *Primacy* and *Individuation*. Individuation is shown by the warship analogy to be an intermediate stage only in the achievement of full operational efficiency for the n-dimensional organism. The highest level of priority is the pursuance of (spiritual) Mission objective.

Furthermore, we perceive that ideal forms relate to *Relationships*. And, that each element or *pole* of the relationship works upon the same Goal but from a complementary and co-operative viewpoint – thus achieving a fine balance. Ideal form can be either prescriptive or proscriptive (or both) concerning limits and bounds of behaviour, resources, goals, and behaviour – just the things that Jung shunned.

IN CONCLUSION

To conclude this monograph, I must begin by giving a very brief elaboration of each of the words in its title (every word has a significance that is, perhaps, more clearly explicit in the following Epilogue).

The word 'Jung' reflects the fact that – after many years (decades) of deliberation (and trial and error) – I have decided that Jungian theory is the best 'gateway' to the various '_roads_' towards understanding and consequent action. When 'corrected' (in the statistical sense of re-orientation of 'skewness'), Jungian constructs are elevated to a rank equalling Plato's.

The word 'Revisited' is an expansion of this in regard of my current approach and its 'perspective'. It is _epitheoretic_ and it aims to be integrative. I have made every effort – when making use of concepts from all individual systems of thought – _never_ to go so deeply into any that my thesis becomes 'entrapped' within it.

This having been said, I search for Truth in Jungian theory that goes deeper than the modes of Judgment and Perception, and their corresponding functions. Those functions of Sensation, Thinking, Intuiting, and Feeling, excellent though they are, do not take an investigator deeply enough into the question, 'Judgment and Perception of What'?

For example, Jung's ideas take one into Experience, through Nature, Nurture, and Environment, but they stop dead at the point of entry into such philosophical matters as Teleology and Ontology. This is fair enough because Jung declared his allegiance to the Christian faith, but to anyone _outside_ that faith (or inside it, for that matter) his assertions are 'skewed'.

As for 'Refreshed', the 'refreshment' comes from the revisit and it derives from critical adherence to the thoughts of 'Jung, the Empiricist' and the 'purging' (for want of a better word) of the thoughts of 'Jung, the doctor of the Soul'. Jung really believed that his talents lay in that direction.

As is evident in Part One of the monograph, I have made every effort to be utterly _rigorous_ in all of these activities. However, I cannot speak for any aspect of my personality and character which is from '_outside_' the materiality of my body. I have done my best – and, in saying that, I am referring to phenomena categorized under _Mysticism_ but (apparently) open to _Factual Experience_.

And, in this, I seem to have a considerable advantage over Jung. I am sure of this, so far as any statistician will make that affirmation, at least in regard of our relative Natures, Nurtures, and Environments. And, I assert this because – concerning my identity – I was a completely 'blank slate' when I made my first, rational, action decision.

It follows from this that, at that moment, I had no notion of self-interest and only the notion of 'Other-interest'. Moreover, there was no emotional content at all. The Epilogue gives an account of my 'growth' in those departments.

This small book, so far as I can make it so, contains no 'hidden agenda', no 'items of faith' in its arguments as distinct from 'items of belief', no conjecture in place of logic, no claims as to 'the Truth' that are unsupported by specifications of 'context and theme', and no call upon 'experience' that has not been subjected to the most rigorous examination and analysis.

In short, it presents some of the contents of the history of my search for *Understanding* of myself and my environment. More precisely, the monograph contains *Information* which I feel (or my 'daimon' feels) could be of use to others and which will be unavailable to them unless it is aired.

I have no axe to grind other than this sole objective – except perhaps (with a rare show of sentiment) to make some small repayment to a field of human endeavour (Science) which has been very kind and generous to me.

My 'story', so to speak, is presented as such in the following personal Epilogue, and any conjecture that I have made during its enactment has been in regard of contributions made to it by my personal circumstances through my Nature and my Nurture. For instance, my scientific 'life' is entwined with my so-called 'world-line', and I am not sure whether Nature or Nurture led me to this (or both).

I can give specific examples. My natural reaction to authority and my strong heterosexuality arise quite clearly in my genetic inheritance from my mother. Fortunately, they appear to be perfectly counter-balanced by the genetic inheritance from my father. This seems as clear as the physiological inheritance, facially, from my father, and grandfather, and possibly my great-grandfather. [My senior son groans at his prospects!]

The first coherent situation that I can recall – in accordance with Piaget's chronicle of development – was about the age of three in which, as I have said, 'I' made my first rational action-decision. It was a simple decision 'to do' or 'not to do' based purely on my reading of the situation – nothing else. I made the right decision and this was subsequently verified.

Later in my development – around puberty or pre-puberty – I made a similar decision of the same type and, after reflective analysis, I have reasons for supposing it to be correct, too. This time, however, there was no prior evaluation process and it involved a completely sudden switch from 'doing' to 'not doing' without pre-meditation.

I like the phrase, 'Intimations of Subordinacy', not only because of its link with poetry but also because it seems to capture my subsequent growth to maturity. Over the subsequent six years or so the number of these occasions increased, as did their importance in the social and sociological scene.

The crux came when my conscious identity (let us call it the Ego) forced its Will over whatever was causing resistance (in the ordinary sense of the word). The experience seemed very, very *physical*, yet, surely, it was all in my mind? And, the occasion could only be called *auspicious* because it led me a long way down the wrong road (which didn't seem so, at the time).

In this, I claim to be perfectly 'normal' or 'ordinary'. A number of clerics, for example, have reported that following 'retrospective analysis' they have found that miracles happen when they pray and do not happen when they do not pray. And, this phenomenon extends into Natural Theology.

In all other things, in fact, normalcy seems to apply; and I wish for no more. One of my proud boasts has been that 'I never make the same mistake more than half-a-dozen times'. And, at school, I was inordinately pleased at having the sports master say, 'Well done'. The same kind of feelings are evoked when a little boy calls me Mate, or a little girl brings me into her awareness – briefly – with a lovely (and innocent) smile. Or, when a fellow sportsman says, 'Good shot'.

But, I have little respect for those who allow – purposely or deliberately – matters of faith to sway their writings unduly. In these things, I admit to being disrespectful to my betters. We must have *comparative* and *epitheoretic* studies, of course, but, in my opinion, we are completely swamped by a sea of dissemblance, misrepresentation, misinformation, disinformation, over-zealous libertarianism, and 'economies with the truth', all of which are 'politically correct', of course.

It really will not do.

However, as Sherrington might have said, by taking this on one is confronting fearsome enemies. In comparison with the diabolerie seemingly involved, von Bertalanffy's wonderful creation, *the social Leviathan,* becomes just a great big 'pussy-cat'. C.S. Lewis seems to have had the right ideas.

We may have 'Roads' to Reality and 'Comprehensive' Reality, and their like, but the dangers besetting humanity are part of the 'Visible Reality' described by Lewis in which the social Leviathan is just a small paring tool in the limbs of that Hideous Strength.

This is the ground covered by the Jung-Plato paradigm – that of 'Visible Reality' and of 'Determinant Reality' – which favours both Action and 'Enaction' in the realm of *material* bodies. Enaction referring to the acting out of a prescribed 'story' rather than Emergence.

Jung perceives that Evil is 'determinant reality', professing not to know how to 'deal' with it, and Plato assures us that only a philosopher or a lover (with some knowledge of philosophy) may achieve the level of divinity. The paradigm 'mechanizes' this (in the manner of MacKay) by having Love as an 'Agent of Change'.

To put this into perspective, the process of mechanizing Love is extremely well covered by Ethel Person's *categories*, by Rollo May's inclusion of an *action imperative*, by Robert Solomon's *classification of emotions*, and by Manfred Clynes's contributions to the *experience* and *communication* of emotion.

In all such respects, therefore, a very neat and pleasing discrimination is drawn between so-called 'items of faith' and the very great men – of all religious persuasions – who have set out exemplary patterns of behaviour for us to follow in the material world. And, but for one more point, I think that this is a good place for me to stop.

My final observation is that the level of these malignant entities is, fortunately, beyond our reach; but even a 'friendly', comparatively low-level encounter with, say, the force and power of an 'archetype' is an awesome event that imprints itself upon one's mind-set and inspires emotions and inclinations utterly foreign to one's nature and nurture. Trust me, I speak from experience!?

Finis

SEMI-AUTOBIOGRAPHICAL EPILOGUE

C. G. Jung expressed great admiration for the philosopher, Plato; and the eminent Jungian, W.E.R. Mons, refers to Jung's update of Plato's ideas. My allusion to a 'Jung-Plato' paradigm is not, therefore, untoward. And, I maintain, such a paradigm is particularly Timely.

Little updating of Plato's notions is necessary. Roger Penrose, a current working mathematician espouses 'mathematical Platonism' and the term 'soul-mate' is understood by most people and used by many more. The illustrious mathematician of his day, A.N. Whitehead, remarked that 'the history of Philosophy is nothing but a series of footnotes to Plato'.

A point worth making, here, is that mathematical Platonism has _everything_ fixed and permanent. This means that the introduction of _anything_ pertaining to Time has to be in terms of a 'wavefront' of energy, force, power, activation or whatever, passing through this fixed and permanent ground.

Although mathematical Platonism avoids the 'messiness' of quantum theory, interaction between fields of information and fields of force converts Potential into Real as it happens in a computer [and, of course, this process is pertinent to Time – as are all 'processes'). And, mathematical Platonism addresses, in particular, Plato's concept of 'Ideal Form', contained within a special realm of 'etheriality' introduced by Roger Penrose.

In respect of this notion, we encounter (a) the need expressed by L. von Bertalanffy for correct _categorization_ of constructs, and (b) the need expressed by Elizabeth Bates (and by C.S. Peirce) for conveying meaning of terms by the specification of apposite _contexts_ and _themes_. And, thereby, we return to Plato and Penrose.

If we view the former's 'mind-set' (i.e. ideology or collection of ideas) in terms of real-time _computer systems_ rather than computing machines, we arrive at a different _category_ for the notion of 'etheriality' in regard of life-processes. Consider, for instance, Dr. Penrose's favourite little unicellular organism, the paramecium.

Purely for example, we might envisage a distinction between a region just 'outside' space and time (in which the sets of ideal forms and their inter-relationships are stored) and that part just 'inside' space-time, i.e. the 'quantum vacuum', (which maintains and controls the so-called 'working space' of the central processing unit of the system and its special registers).

We can appreciate that Plato's ideas are coherent in that scenario, and we can even _add_ to mathematical Platonism in such respects by introducing the scheme of thought advanced by Donald MacKay, which he called 'Comprehensive Realism' and which featured the literal 'embodiment' of a mathematical formula.

Donald MacKay's contribution to our understanding of the human mind has been called 'the mechanization of mind-like processes', in which the physiological processes of the living body are replicated (speaking loosely) by processes in a computer. My, separate and independent, expansion of Comprehensive Reality is to include the 'replication' of _psychological_ processes.

It is far more difficult than this to accommodate the original ideas of Jung within mathematics and/or mathematical physics as they pertain to computer systems. It can be done – at least in regard of certain key or pivotal issues. However, certain groundwork has to be done before any start can be made.

First, it must be recognized and accepted that – on his own repeated admission – all Jung's valued concepts had been formulated in the years preceding, say, the mid-1920s. Second, that during that period, and thereafter, his _nature_, _nurture_, and _circumstances_ were such that any move towards accommodation must include some degree of scientific analysis of his mentality (i.e. his 'mind-set') and his personality and 'character'.

By this, I mean reference to Freud and to Rank (in a comparative study made by Ruth Munroe), and references to the likes of Ethel Spector Person and Rollo May (both of whom might be called 'psychiatrists of Love'). I include with these, comments by Jungians about Jung's ideology which are critical and not always justified or acceptable.

I can improve on this by referring to six Victorians who between them ushered in a philosophical change from 'the Age of Individualism' to the 'Age of Relationism' (which obtains today regarding the physical universe which is held to contain only relationships and fields).

The assertions of three psychotherapists and the arguments of a matching _triage_ of mathematicians reflect the period of transition, as follows:

Jung asserted that 'the goal of psychic development is the _Self_'

Freud conceived of a libidinous 'force' driving one to fix upon some 'Other'

Rank saw the Will of the whole Personality to be focussed on the 'Other'

Cantor demonstrated that Infinity consists of Transfinite structures/relations

Ouspensky introduced 'intuitional logic' covering 'both A and Not-A'

Whitehead coupled experience with the basic organization of Plato's ideas.

Today, well into the 21st-century, there is almost a plethora of reputable mathematicians adding their own individual 'footnotes' to Plato. Such a 'weight of opinion' can become, in principle, a 'weight of _evidence_' because (as I show in Part One) the value of opinion as evidence can be quantized, accumulated, and evaluated. This (as I illustrate in part Three) is best done epitheoretically and by computer or, better, a computer network.

Be that as it may, there are three modern mathematicians among them who, I'm sure, would have found favour with Plato (say at the proverbial 'dinner party'). They are, in no particular order, Roger Penrose, Rudy Rucker, and Donald MacKay; and I nominate them now because their scientific constructs lead directly to an examination of Jungian theory.

In short, the thoughts of Plato, Penrose, and Rucker combine almost impeccably to provide for MacKay's mechanistic embodiment of a mathematical formula as an 'n-dimensional' organism within the physical universe, functioning in both the _material_ realm/level and the _non-material_ realms/levels which subtend the material entities.

MacKay's model describes to perfection two 'Functionaries' covering differing areas of responsibility. One functionary is nominated as 'the Agent', which organizes the processes of the physiological organism, and the other functionary is called 'the Determinator', which is concerned especially with the selection of possible 'action-alternatives'. The Agent provides for the Determinator a variety of possible actions from which to select a preferred action.

The 'MacKay model' is based upon Donald MacKay's so-called mechanization of 'mind-like processes' which was derived from his intimate knowledge of a real-time computer system. And, I know (from working on the same system and a correspondence with him over a number of years) that our understandings of this kind of computer system are identical.

His concept of 'duality without dualism' unifies the thoughts of Victorian, C.S. Sherrington, with the modern, Ernest W. Kent. The former needs no introduction, and the latter is a 'physiological psychologist' and 'psycho-pharmacologist', and they sing very much from the same hymn sheet.

Sherrington would have viewed the Determinator as an 'ultimate pontifical nerve-cell', and Kent expressed his belief that the Determinator function lies in the 'feed-foreword' processes of the fore-brain. Kent appears to be a trifle confused in his computer analogies, but that is of no consequence.

Not only does the MacKay model locate the action in the physiological materiality of the brain, but it also roots so-called mystical phenomena with brain activity as it is perceivable through electroencephalographic recordings. This is described in the two works by William Johnston, _The Inner Eye of Love_ and _Silent Music._

To balance this, we have Ouspensky's so-called 'intuitive logic', and the two specific organismal functions provided by Jung (Intuition and Feeling) which, when paired together, afford us with the _experiential knowledge_ that goes a step beyond Ouspensky's logic (and is quantifiable and evidential).

As experiential knowledge is the stuff of mysticism, we are led to consider the 'Road of the East' and the 'Road of the West', only to find that they cover much the same terrain rather than converge towards an end-point. For example, the Sino-Asiatic yogic tradition is built upon five thousand years of the rational analysis of phenomenological experience.

In fact, both 'Roads' are in accordance with the notions and criteria of Plato. From the West, the change in level or scale descends to the _smallest parts of the material, i.e. 'quarks'_, and beyond that into the realms of Plato's _superurgoi_, i.e. demi-gods or other 'Causal' entities. And, coming the other way we proceed from the so-called 'Causal plane' up into the material realm of atoms and molecules, i.e. _manifestations._

It is noteworthy that Jung's concept of a 'Life Force' containing two principles, the Male and the Female, is a very close match to the Hindu yogic concept of a Life Energy releasing – only in the physical universe – the principles of the Yin and the Yang. Jung was aware of this.

The difficulty with Jung, however, lies in his insistence that _Personality_ is lodged in a system that is separate and distinct from the material realm. Probably, he would have seen no difficulty with this, and would have 'located' the system in some 'extra' dimensions of the physical universe.

The radical flaw in such an arrangement is that Personality – exactly as he portrayed it – can be attributed to _any_ material system, living, non-living, or 'hybrid, pursuing a purposeful organismal course in a real-time situation. This I demonstrate in Part Two by showing that the real-time computer system of an operational warship has all the characteristics of Personality.

In a nutshell, it can be said that the MacKay model is derivable from the concepts and precepts of particle physics and of mysticism. Or, that the model is consonant with Plato. Or, simply, that Jungian theory must be changed. I have met with a number of Jungians, and, therefore, know from experience that their dispositions differ – including willingness to change.

My first observation is that 'the warship analogy', as it might be called, is likely to completely misconceived as an 'over-strong defence mechanism'. It is, of course, no such thing. Provided that the warship is from a civilized country, its sole purpose is the defence and welfare of the Other. Indeed, the authority of _Command_ carries with it the expectation of Self-Sacrifice.

My second observation is that the accompanying notion of tiers or echelons of intercommunication between warships, under the appropriate 'centre' for Command and Control and Communications, is very well-liked by Jungians. Especially, as the higher levels are, or should be, Normative and Deontic (and, as we have seen, Political).

There is more to it than this, however. For example, the 'Jungian problematic' disappears. The goal of development for the organism changes from 'Self' to 'Other'; and _Individuation_ becomes as it is in the warship's Command function, namely to achieve knowledge and mastery of 'Self' so as to attain best operational performance for the organism.

In terms of a physical universe composed only of relationships and fields, the elegant simplicity of the MacKay model and its necessity become enhanced. Amid a teeming myriad of relationships, most of which are false, spurious, misleading, etc., all injurious to our best interests, the only 'truth' lies between the _affinitive poles_ of a 'mechanistically embodied bi-variable function'. Metaphorically speaking, everything else is 'winnowed out'.

In this kind of relationship, 'Determinator M' and 'Determinator F' are the poles, and the _Animus/Anima_ Function of each pole is 'guided' by the knowledge of its own pole and its own pole's recollection of former union. This is not only exquisite symmetry, but it also captures the Yin and Yang principles co-operating with each other as in the Hindu yogic tradition.

To put it another way, n Platonism, each Anima/Animus is governed by its pole's recollection of former union and is aided by its perception of existing and available action alternatives. In principle, it can actually see the 'Anticipated Whole Other'.

In short, the Anima/Animus function is _Real_. The 'Anticipated Whole Other' is a real thing – it is a Target or, if you like, a Mission Objective. It is most definitely _NOT_ a stochastically gathered accumulation of features of real women gathered together to furnish an entirely fictive image of a woman that is disposable after use.

Our belief is justified because the whole of Mystical Knowing is to do with the variety of levels and kinds open to an affinitive relationship of this kind. The words of Hiroshi Motoyama and of William Johnston pay tribute to these wonders and splendours. They boost our own experiences, but, to put things into proportion, we should regard relationships, _en masse._

However, before going into further detail in those respect, it behoves us to return, first, to the recent notions of Danah Zohar and, second, to the notions held, some two hundred and fifty years earlier, by philosopher, David Hume (mentioned particularly by Rudy Rucker). They most apposite _and_ significant.

Danah Zohar, it will be remembered, makes both the identification required by Plato of 'the smallest parts of matter' and 'that which is "non-matter" '. The disjunction she offers is, essentially, that between the varieties of 'quarks' and 'leptons'. However, in regard of material men and women, she pitches it at a higher level, i.e. the distinction between particles called 'Fermions' (matter) and particles called 'Bosons' (non-matter).

The point that Ms. Zohar wants to make is the fact that, in her phraseology, 'We _Are_ our relationships'. And, her argument is based upon wave/particle 'complementarity', which obtains _at that level_. At the deeper level, one encounters the influences and effects of the Life Force and its principles (in the physical universe) of Femininity and Masculinity.

At the deeper levels, therefore, our relationships are more elective _and_ more eclectic – depending upon one's perspective. As for Hume, without digressing too much into his naturalism and empiricism, there are three features that pertain especially to the 'Zoharian' or 'Platonic' disjunction or interface. The distinction is one of level.

The first feature is that, in a world of relationships, contexts, and fields (and their organizational details), Hume's belief that 'there is no logical bridge between fact and value' is completely untenable. In contradistinction, Hume's view that 'perceptions are primary' seems unchallengeable – at least to evolutionary psychologists.

It is Hume's third point, in regard of the divisibility of a human organism's perceptual field, which immediately captures our attention. For our benefit, Rucker construes this into the concept of our space-time 'being supplemented by an additional dimension of _scale_' (his italics). And, acceptance of this proposition takes us immediately, and full blown, into the Realm of the 'Experiencing of Knowledge' (i.e. my suggested 'Quartic Organum').

In one bound, metaphorically speaking, we perceive that our relationships _do_ have to be ordered, evaluated and prioritized. Indeed, that is an essential element in the MacKay model. And, because of the encephalization of Personality, so is the arranging of and discriminating between emotional 'ties', 'bonds', 'needs', 'desires', 'obligations', and 'facts' in our relationships.

In short, Plato, Jung, and MacKay are united in Mysticism in a way that follows from the concepts of Cantor and Ouspensky and Priestley. Jung perceived this, but his nature, nurture, and circumstances forbade its acceptance. Yet, as Priestley explained to us, the Experience is there for us all to comprehend – Everyman (and his Anima) and Everywoman (and her Animus). We _are_ our relationships – but some are better than others.

And so, we have finally arrived at that which Jung tried to hide, a _realistic_ appreciation of the Growth of mutual personal love. Avoiding the theory-loaded terminology of both Jung and William Johnston, there is at base _carnal_ love. Then, _Romantic_ love and _Devotional_ love, and finally, at the approach to divinity, there is _Sapientia_.

As William Johnston points out, these kinds of Love are neither necessarily sequential nor mutually exclusive. Following Rucker and Ouspensky, each stretches 'from here to Infinity', and this can be imagined and portrayed by taking the dimensions of Scale as an abscissa, and the amount of 'completeness' or 'indwelling' or '_Re-union_' of each relationship as the ordinate.

This actually has much resonance with Ouspensky's notion of _dimensional time_, and Rucker gives this due attention in his book, THE FOURTH DIMENSION AND HOW TO GET THERE. My immediate interest, however, is to relate the concept to an irrational and transcendental mathematical _growth function_ which, to my mind, has more apposite contextual cogency.

The function to which I refer is one that I have used before - as I have described in a number of papers (in the _Journal of Naval Science_). Although it is a commonly used growth function, the Logistic function appears to possess properties particularly suited for the circumstances obtaining in the treatment of Scale as a dimension.

Having made remarks about Jung's nature, nurture, and circumstances, and being able to match him on the matter of Visions and Personifications, I am obliged to indicate some key aspects of my own nature, nurture, and circumstances over my lifetime, so far. As might be expected, they are in stark contrast.

For example, I think it fair to say that the first five years of my life – up to my starting at Infant school – saw me as a rational being within a 'vacuum' of experience, ratiocination, and emotion. This vacuum obtained, during those years, entirely on 'the wrong side of the tracks', although a very acute and perceptive friend once observed that I 'grew up with a foot either side of the tracks'.

This, I can amplify. It was due almost entirely (in my opinion) due to a complete contrast between the cultural outlook and values, respectively, of my two sets of grandparents – although, of course, genetics *did* play its part in furnishing my dispositions, tastes, and *possibly* my values.

Eight decades of developing my *Persona* left me almost fully equipped to deal with the necessities of survival and the development of analytical skills concerning both people and situations. It left me, however, completely _feral_ in my attitude to life and to the world about me; and it was at this point, I felt myself elevated to Sapientia.

My children, who don't pull their punches, refer to my Damascene conversion, but although the conversion was real enough it did not seem to have a religious content. In terms of the MacKay model, I had moved in consciousness from being an Agent to being a Determinator.

Better than this is Plato's concept of the Charioteer. This entity was (loosely) the Determinator part of a three-part entity, of which the White horse was Good and the Black horse was Bad. My conversion, so to speak, was equivalent to the Charioteer's taming of the Black horse and then being able to use its power.

There are other interpretations in terms of degrees of mystical union, merger, indwelling, etc., but, for me, the conversion has given me the power to join _facts_ with _values_. 'I' no longer relates to me; in fact it no longer has any meaning. Neither does 'consciousness' hold meaning. Meaning does not obtain in the extra dimensions of the physical universe.

It is the knowledge obtained in these dimensions that endows our material bodies with the ability to connect facts with values. But, the material bodies, the conscious egos, have also changed. The use of the Persona, for example, is regarded as an unworthy form of deceit. The 'I' you see is the 'I' you get. 'Worthiness' has become a measure of value – in complete opposition to the notion of 'patience becoming an asset'.

Perhaps, Williamson and Pearse were right to invent their own vocabulary. A realm of 'Quality', surely can hardly be bettered. Or, one of 'Aesthesia' to accommodate *feelings*, which are associated with *eclectivity* in the dimension *Memory-Will*. The notion of 'Appositeness' gives one, in their scheme, the ability to weight Facts with Values, all governed by specifications of contexts and themes.

Williamson and Pearse make it quite clear that are shading the meanings of concepts discussed in the mystical dimensions of East and of West. And, of course, they avoid the dangers of building in obfuscating elements of faith, superstition, hope, frustration, spite, envy, and their like.

This takes me quite naturally to *my* Visions and Personifications, and these are sufficiently close to Jung's reports of such things for me to think of hypnagogic imagery processes, 'higher' and 'lower', corresponding to MacKay's model and to the Jung-Plato paradigm of which it is a part.

I can *Explain* my experiences in this domain _only_ by the Jung-Plato paradigm. Some of them have effected a change in my attitudes, perspectives, motivation, that is truly *Ineffable* and momentous. So far as I can ascertain, those descriptors have left my Judgment and Perception completely unaffected.

Within the limitation of ineffability, I can also *Describe* certain individual instances in terms of likelihoods and the kernels of <u>*fact*</u> which each contains. In regard of things like William Johnston's descriptions of Mysticism (and union, merger, indwelling, etc.) this has importance. However, of even more importance ontologically are the underlying <u>*mathematical*</u> foundations.

A natural return to the world of mathematics for me is by way of the Logistic growth function, about which I wrote a number of papers (*The Journal of Naval Science*) in the 1960s. The function and its properties seem particularly appealing in view of an 'Axis of Scale' (along a *dimension of Scale)* and of *Completeness and Quality* (along an axis of *mystical Knowledge* at right angles to it).

In this respect, the term coined by Williamson and Pearse seems particularly appropriate. The term is, 'Aesthesia', and it involves, among other things, the notion (advanced by Ouspensky as intuitive logic) of the 'synthesis of the "Self" with the "Not-Self" '.

I had vague ideas of using the properties of the Logistic (which I had demonstrated decades before) to reflect the 'Sino-Asiatic' qualities of the paradigm in terms of Plato and 'the One and the Many' described assiduously by Rudy Rucker – after all, the view from the East and Middle-East is often reflected in terms of hydrodynamics of rivers, seas, etc.

This was accompanied by the similarities that I thought I could see in the concepts being advanced by Roger Penrose of mathematical concepts such as 'twistor sheaf cohomology', Riemannian space, and other features leading to his notion of Strong Determinism which fits, it seems, impeccably with Comprehensive Reality.

This train of thought seemed to be well on course when I read the assertion by Rucker that 'Attempts to analyse the phenomenon of consciousness and self-awareness rationally appear to lead to infinite regresses' (1982, p.51).

That statement, coming from an author deemed to have brought together 'every aspect of mathematical infinity from the infinitesimals of non-standard analyses to the transfinite numbers of Cantor and the surreal numbers of Conway', and its description, are both in error.

Neither '*Infinity and he Mind...*' nor '*The fourth Dimension...*' contains a very important and highly-regarded element in Ouspensky's *Tertium Organum* which completely negates the concept of infinite regression.

Ouspensky conceived of the intuitive logic that couples together the categorizations 'I' and 'Not-I', that is to say, the categories of 'Self' and of 'Other' which were the root of the Jungian 'problematic'. This conjunction within the same category, i.e. set, runs parallel with 'synthesis of the "Self" with the "Not-Self" ' in a higher realm of Aesthesia conjectured by Williamson and Pearse (p. 205).

We are clearly in important waters over such matters, and the idea of grimly, determinedly, and unsentimentally labouring towards 'Improvement' throughout the kind of 'Recurrence' described by Gurdjieff and, then, his disciple Ouspensky, was in line with this notion of infinite regression _and_ with many celebrated Jungians who, naturally, welcomed the notion of Self-Improvement through hard work and suffering.

Pleased with the growing harmony between the world of mathematics, portrayed by Roger Penrose, and the 'J-P paradigm', I become somewhat concerned about the balance and the depth of Rudy Rucker's 'take' (i.e. perspective) on the ideology of P.D. Ouspensky. I can give several instances.

The obvious example, I suppose, is the discrepancy between the title, '_The Fourth Dimension..._' and Ouspensky's concept of a three dimensional Time analogous to three dimensional Space. And, another one, of equal significance, is Rucker's apparent focusing upon Recurrence and infinite regression.

Although I feel that the 'Logistic function over the Axis of Scale' model would have been adequate, This is both dwarfed by and subsumed within the works of J.B. Priestley and of J.G. Bennett which are contained in Priestley's _Man and Time_. And, I agree completely with its reviewers – and more. J.G. Bennett was a Jungian.

In fact, I believe (a word I seldom use) that Priestley and Bennett have made a _monumental_ contribution to our conception of Existence. The former writes his personal _Experience_ into the J-P paradigm, together with ESP (Extra-Sensory Perception), and the latter effectively turns MacKay's Comprehensive Reality into an _all-subsuming_ mathematical formula that was presented to the Royal Society.

The twin concepts of Relationism and 'encephalized Personality' eliminate the Jungian problematic and enhance the Jung-Plato paradigm, but the key, pivotal and profound, thinking in all of this comes from J.B. Priestley and his friend, the business-man and mathematician, J.G. Bennett, as is 'delightfully' reported in Priestley's _Man and Time_.

Jung described himself as a functionary in two contrasting ways which interJtwine throughout _Memories, Dreams, Reflections_. The first of these is that of an observer who accepts that ultimate truths may well be inaccessible to human thought and who throws out ideas which are not necessarily consistent or coherent with each other.

The second description of himself as a functionary is when he claims to be a 'doctor of the soul' who has personal experiences of God and dismisses the living stream of Evolution as 'biological turmoil' – completely ignoring the implications of Relationism set out by Freud.

To arrive, finally, at the Jung-Plato paradigm we must follow 'Jung – the Empiricist' rather than 'Jung – the soul-doctor'. Thus, we move on from the encephalized brain/mind and the reified Animus/Anima to address Jung's interpretation of the Sino-Asiatic model of karma and reincarnation.

This needs correction – as is to be seen in _Man and His Symbols_ – but little change is needed because it is achieved simply by re-aligning the four functions of perception and judgment, exactly as they were set out originally by Jung. The pairing becomes (a) Sensation-Thinking and (b) Sensing-Intuiting, and it brings judgment and Perception precisely into line with Cantor and Ouspensky.

There are deeper consequences than this, however, which I *must* mention before moving on. For example, the regrouping of the functions not only *explains* Jung's exclusion of 'emotional ties' but it also *accentuates* his failure to consider 'emotional *bonds*', such as those in the natural quaternion (i.e. Parent, Offspring, Sibling, Other).

The change of pairing also rationalizes and decouples (or uncouples) *Sex* and *Love*. After all, 'Sex' is all about SENSATION and THINKING about it. In contradistinction, 'Love' is all about INTUITION and FEELING. And, we can even take this further – into MYSTICISM and MYSTICAL KNOWLEDGE.

By this I mean that certain concepts or constructs become joined up or relativized at the highest level (within the physical union). Sapientia, for example, is a system STATE. At that level, NOESIS is mystical knowledge – defined as being obtained in a realm 'beyond' mathematics (Blackburn, p. 263). And, Ouspensky's *intuitional logic* (Tertium Organum) is supplemented by the *experience* of knowledge within a relationship, namely my suggested 'Quartic Organum'.

Thus, we move into the realm of Mysticism as it is described by William Johnston but without the input from him of religious dogma. By our consideration exclusively of the physical universe we have arrived at the lowest Realm of the Sino-Asiatic model and its notions on mystical relationships in terms of human experience and of *extra* dimensions of Space, Time, and beyond Space-Time.

This brings me to my most recent experience, which is utterly different from all the others because it involves an encounter with a different kind of *Being* ('entity' is far too tame a word). The 'Presence' was not only part of 'my' story (why else would it intervene?) but also 'outside' in the sense of the 'non-locality' which so intrigues Roger Penrose.

The Being was aware of my twinned motivations. One goal being 'completion' of the production of this monograph in the material realm. The other goal being 'completion' at the much higher, 'Sapientic', level and in the Platonic mode of 'Re-Union'. And, it was awesome. So awe-inspiring that, although it identified itself, I could not assimilate the words that were being 'boomed', 'roared', 'seared', into my mind. It seemed truly ineffable.

On reflection, the Being was on a 'higher' authoritative and ontological level. It may have been an 'archetypal form' of some kind. Or, a 'worldly representation' of a minor divinity. Or a demiurge. Or (from the Sino-Asiatic model) the masked raw power of the Yin. Or, its equivalent in Jungian theory, aka Eros. Or, the Hindu yogic 'Crown Chakra'.

The imperative coming from the Being, which was operating at (I surmise) the 'causal level, was in natural language and was couched in terms completely pertinent to my twinned goals. It said, almost verbatim, 'Don't waste time mooning over Rosamunda, concentrate on publishing the monograph'.

And so I did – I had no choice. What information lay in that imperative? And, what Purpose? It seems to have been very necessary, with hindsight, because for six weeks after Christmas I was incapable of conducting any kind of printing arrangements, And, these had been done. In fact, the publishing date is approaching rapidly and it marks (or caps) eighty-five years of Growth and Analysis.

I can provide a possible explanation in the context of the Being. A month or two earlier, I had received one of Jung's hints from the Unconscious, as I thought, which I interpreted as merely a statement of the situation obtaining. I perceived no action imperative in the communiction. If I *had* misinterpreted the message, then perhaps a higher level authority might have stepped in. However, in that case, there would be implications for both me and my project. Time may tell.

My surmises about the 'ontological' levels may not be mutually exclusive. If we examine my 'mechanization quartet' of the preceding section – Person, May, Solomon, Clynes – then we find that, if Love *is* an agent of change, then we are all enacting differing 'stories'. For example, this monograph seeks to present Truth free of 'clutter'. So does poetry.

I suspect, however, that Omar Khayyam's story has a 'sub-plot' different from mine. Through his relationship with his Beloved (with his 'other pole') Omar reaches a quality of expression (pace Fitzgerald) indicating his 'destiny'. In *my* polar sub-plot, I am moved by the need (a desperate need) to link Action with Emotion (and with Experience) in revealing Truth.

It seems likely, therefore, that in an affinitive relationship both poles, when the Yin and Yang principles *manifest poles as* people, the relationship has to do with karma rather than being fixed into a recurring sub-plot.   And, in that respect, it may be easier to understand Love as a universal by referring to the Logistic function and remembering that in the Jung-Plato paradigm 'stories' may be re-enacted any number of times.

And, continuing in that vein, I can think of no better way of finishing this monograph than by quoting Donald McCrimmon MacKay, himself. He writes (1980, p. 101) on Death

'What it cannot do, however, is to remove me from all possibility of *re-embodiment* by my Creator if he should so will it.'

The Last Word

Anthony Stevens makes exactly the same point as I do in this rather large monograph (100, 000 words). He believes it possible that the 'new breed' of evolutionary psychologists will, one day, produe a form of 'evolutionary psychotherapy'.   And, he believes, will be undogmatic and open-minded.

This is my argument.   What could be more existential, for example, than mechanistic embodiment in a comprehensive Reality? This is a Jungian concept (e.g.

Archetypes and Ideal Forms), but Existence embraces far more than this – as Jung himself pointed out frequently.

As Rollo May, the _existentialist_ psychotherapist, points out, reality seems to have 'the ontological character' of negative-positive polarity. He indicates the error in the famous sentence of Descartes, 'I think, therefore, I am'. What happens in human experience is 'I conceive-I can-I will-I am', and this links intentionality with vitality, i.e. the determination of 'I will make it so'.

We see that a putative system of evolutionary psychotherapy is (would be) part of a larger existential system. Such a system would be, by definition, epitheoretic, and this is precisely the point at which countless Jungians have already failed. They have not been able to extricate their cognition from the theory in which it is embedded. (Steven Pinker makes the same error – see the Bibliography).

Anthony Stevens follows suit. He identifies the qualities of being undogmatic and open-minded with Jung – and who would challenge that? But, a further identification of the qualities is with another qualitative feature or category, to which Jung undoubtedly belonged but which is also epitheoretic and eclectic.

Indeed, the term to which I refer has a variety of meanings, of which only some are identifiable with Jung. I am sure that the categorization of Jung, accordingly, would be varied among my readers. Also, that some of the categories would be utterly repugnant to dedicated Jungians. Nevertheless, I ask them bravely to bite the bullet and to consider seriously, from that viewpoint, the term, HUMANITY.

FINIS

ANNOTATED BIBLIOGRAPHY

Nearly every book listed in this Bibliography is on, or has been on, the shelves of my study, and the selection is highly personal – always guided by my desire for rigour. The two large establishments at which I worked (ARL and ASWE) had large and efficient libraries and, in its early days, the RNSS and, then, the Scientific Civil Service operated highly organized Information Services.

At the small laboratory (RNPL), when I was working in experimental psychology, I was always up-to-date by working from the USA's current Handbook of Experimental Psychology – my wife was the Librarian!?

Armstrong, 'john' (2002), *conditions of love*, Norton, USA.

Arnold, A. (1998), *Inner Scripts*. Waterweaver Press, Montrose, Scotland.

Arnold Arnold (1992), *THE CORRUPTED SCIENCES*, Paladin (HarperCollins.

[From the front cover to the back cover, this book is useful. For example, it contains eleven pages on the dimensionality of Time, And. it cites two of 'my' authors on that subject, namely J.B.Priestley and G.J. Whitrow – it is the only one, out of more than a dozen books on Time, to do this]

Augustine, St. (1969), *THE CONFESSIONS OF ST. AUGUSTINE*, Airmont, NY.

Ayer, A.J. (1976), *The Central Questions of Philosophy*, Pelican/Penguin.

-------- (1972), *The Problem of Knowledge*, Pelican/Penguin.

Ball, Philip (2001), *stories of the invisible*, OUP [of wide potential use]

Barrow, John (1992), *Pi in the Sky*, OUP.

[Penrose, Plato, and mathematical Intuition]

Bates, E. (1976), *Language and Context*: *the acquisition of Pragmatics*.

Academic Press, Inc. (LONDON) Ltd.

Bentov, I. (1979), *STALKING THE WILD PENDULUM,* Fontana/Collins, Glasgow.

Berne, Eric (1978), *What Do You Say After You Say Hello?*, Corgi.

Berne, Eric (1968), *Games People Play*, Penguin books.

von Bertalanffy, L. (1967), *Robots, Men and Minds: Psychology in the Modern World*. George Braziller, New York.

---------(1973), *General System Theory*. Penguin University Books.

Bettelheim, Bruno (1983), *Freud & Man's Soul*, Chatto & Windus, London.

Bird, Graham (1972), *Philosophical Tasks,,,,* Hutchinson.

Blackburn, Simon (1994), *THE OXFORD DICTIONARY OF PHILOSOPHY*, OUP.

Blakemore, Colin (1991), *The Mind Machine*, BBC Books (Classics), London.

Blakeslee, S. & Ramachandran, V.S. (2005), *PHANTOMS IN THE BRAIN…,,*

       Harper Perennial.

     [Abnormality and normality in mystical experience, the temporal lobe in religion, the varieties of religious experience, different kinds of Self, consonance with MacKay; Kosslyn, Priestley, etc., but too restricted to be useful.The point is made, however, that the brain areas associated with religious or mystical experience can be used to disprove or to prove the existence of God]

Boden, Margaret, (1978), *Purposive Explanation in Psychology*, Harvester

       Press, England.

Boyer, Carl B. (1991), *A History of Mathematics,* Wiley.

Bono (de), Edward (1979), *The Mechanism of Mind*, Pelican.

Braithwaite, R.B. (1968), *Scientific Explanation…*, CUP.

Braude, S.E. (1986), *The Limits of Influence…,* Routledge & Kegan Paul.

BBC Ed. (1967), *DECISION MAKING*, British Broadcasting Corporation, London.

Brown, J.A.C. (1954), *The Social Psychology of Industry*, Pelican/Penguin.

Buchanan, M. (2002*), small world: uncovering nature's networks*. Weidenfeld

       and Nicholson, London.

Buckley, P. Editor (1988), *ESSENTIAL PAPERS ON PSYCHOSIS*, NY University.

Burt, Cyril, (1962), 'Mind and Consciousness'. In *The Scientist Speculates* by I.   I.J. Good (Ed.), Heinemann, London.

Calvin, W.H. (1997), *HOW BRAINS THINK…,* Weidenfeld & Nicolson, London.

Cantor, G. (1915), *CONTRIBUTIONS TO THE FOUNDIND OF THE THEORY OF*

       TRANSFINITE NUNBERS, Dover Publications, New York.

       [see also Huntington]

Capra, Fritjof, (1979), *THE TAO OF PHYSICS*, Wildwood House, Ltd., London.

--------- (1982), *THE TURNING POINT*, Wildwood House, Ltd., London.

Carter, R. (2002), *CONSCIOUSNESS*, Weidenfeld & Nicolson, U.K.

--------   (1998), *MAPPING THE MIND*, Weidenfeld & Nicolson, London.

Chen Ying Yang (1963), *Elementary Particles*, Princeton University Press.

CAUSALITY

As I intimated at the outset of this book, information on Causality has to be mined – it lies very deep and in many diverse fields. Although it was largely conjectural when Aristotle set it up as a subject for study and development, he would have had reasons for his formulations. And today, nearly three thousand years later, they can be recognized in the operations of a stored program real-time computer system.

His formulations lie beyond computation, beyond individual systems of thought, almost beyond conception, and yet within a few years of advent of computers Donald MacCrimmon Mackay and I, separately and independently, were working upon the kind of system that I have described which furnished the information enabling to make such a claim.

It almost goes without saying that the identification of Aristotle's forms of logic as computer processes will not be found in any one book (apart from this one) but I _can_ point to a number of author who can furnish various simple ideas that can be knitted together with comparative ease. And, I list the major authors below.

To put it baldly, I am referring to a material organism (system) that organized and drives certain of its material parts according to instructions on a pattern of information held within itself on its hardware. Change the pattern, or the 'code' in which it is written, and the smallest change may produce radical results (Motoyama).

The essential point is, I suppose, that the arrival of this kind of computer (real-time, stored program) has changed much of our thinking from conjecture or speculation into facts and models. We can now make sense of so many things. For example, we can align Freud's concept of a 'soul' with MacKay's 'core of self-organization', and both can be associated with Purpose and Motivation under a wide variety of disciplines.

Cyril Burt   Interaction - fields force/information

Joan Wynne Reeves   Aristotle's forms of Causality and Potentiality

Ludwig von Bertalanffy   Open systems – from differential equations to

                                   Mental Health and Cultural Relationships.

Donald MacKay   Characters in Stories   Freedom of Action

                              Self-organization   Mechanistic Embodiment

It is worthy of note that doubts expressed by Margaret A, Boden (1978, p. 152) concerning research programs and testability are resolved completely.   Much more significant, however, is the fact that these concepts of Mind, conceived in an

Individualistic world-attitude, translate impeccably into organisms being 'poles' of a relationship. As Danah Zohar has pointed out, 'We _are_ our relationships'.

In terms of specifics, one envisages even Freud (via Bettelheimer) conceiving of a possible 'soul-mate'. Ludwig von Bertalanffy gives us a teleological pull which has to be pursued amid conflict with the social Leviathan, and Donald MacKay reflecting on how easy it is for organisms (systems) to unite, to merge, and (via Johnston) to indwell.

Chown, Marcus (2001), *THE UNIVERSE NEXT DOOR*, Headline Book

Publishing, Hodder Headline, London.

Clarke, D.D. with Crosland, J. (1985), *ACTION SYSTEMS*, Methuen, London.

COMPUTER _SYSTEMS_

Very few people understand computers deeply enough to comprehend that they are regarded widely as being instruments for 'User Systems' but are systems in their own right. It follows that there are no books on computers or computer systems at the level of the quarks and leptons in particle physics.. And so, I am forced to identify those authors whose ideas are, so to speak, _key_ to any rational and worthy discussion, and those whose notions are _fringe_ at best.

When used by a User System, the purposiveness of that system is reflected in the Computer System, and eventually the function of COMMAND becomes distinguishable from the function of COMMAND SUPPORT. Donald MacKay assigns those functions to 'poles' of an embodied formula which he calls, respectively 'the Determinator' and 'the Agent'. Taking both functionaries together – as an organism – a dozen or so features can be observed which seem to point up the errors in the separate and distinctive approaches of Steven Pinker and of Ernest Kent. They are:

Conversion of Potential into Real

Criticality of information 'bits'

Sherrington's principle of Convergence

The 'core' of self-organization

Activation and suspension of processes

Division of labour (Command support and Command)

Pursuit of same goal

A place for these features in Laszlo's theory

Judgments are made on knowledge obtained heuristically

Fields of Force interacting with Fields of Information

All processes operating within one physical system

Mysticism, ESP, Reincarnation, etc., all through extra dimensions

Against this framework, Kent's philosophy could be adapted to accommodate the features but not Pinker's. There is a striking parallel exists between the succession of pictures obtained by moderns with their fingers on and over a 'smart phone' (or whatever) and the action – described by Popper and Eccles – of a 'searchlight' sweeping over the 'liaison brain'.

Using their terms selectively (thus, altering their argument) we can provide our own argument for the Sino-Asiatic model. (This is permissible, because the major point that Popper and Eccles want to make is that the brain is exquisitely suited for being used as a computer by some external system – which they call variously 'Ego', 'Self', 'Soul', and 'inner self').

The neuronal machinery they see as a 'multiplex of radiating and receiving structures'. The attention of the psyche plays over the whole 'liaison brain' selectively. A 'multiple scanning and probing device' is used to read out from and select from the immense and diverse patterns of activity in the cerebral cortex.

This putative device identifies selected components so that the selected sets of fermions (matter) may be acted upon by the appropriate sets of bosons (non-matter). And readers may remember the 'Zoharian Interface' and my comment about a hand playing a piano.

Popper and Eccles give an example of the kind of mechanism they envisage. It is when the psyche is following a line of thought, or trying to recapture a memory, and the psyche is actively engaged in searching and probing through specially selected zones of neural machinery and so is able to *deflect and mould* the dynamic patterned activities in accord with its desire or interest.

My terminology follows closely that used by Popper and Eccles but it presents a different case. However, it matches the collaboration between brain and psyche described by Sherrington (whom they mention). My point is that the underlying mechanism for these processes, which they hardly mention, are supplied, exactly and fully, by the astral and causal 'bodies' of the Sino-Asiatic model. And, this is an example of what Steven Pinker is rejecting.

The matter leads to an issue which is graver by far, and which demands that I make this entry considerably larger than I had intended. My comment is triggered by statements made by Steven Pinker that savour of shallow thinking and/or incompleteness (just as I found with Mattessich). They are made in *The Blank Slate* (p.224) and they are about Science and the Soul.

With breath-taking effrontery or naivete, Pinker defines the soul as being located in the brain's information-processing activities as sentience, reason, and will. Further, he asserts that the 'intuitive and morally useful' concept of a spirit' simply cannot be reconciled with an evolutionary brain.

I would dearly love to continue my commentary on Pinker's remarks in *The STUFF of Thought* (p. 108), in which he identifies Radical Pragmatism as Pragmatism with no mention of Semiotics or C.S. Peirce, and merely categorizes Elizabeth Bates as belonging to that class. However, this subject may lie within my expertise but it is definitely outside my terms of remit, i.e. Jungian theory. Jung just says Meaning – and that is that.

My disquiet over at least some of Steven Pinker's work can be summed up, as follows. He has hypostatized one composite of dubious metaphysical assertions and has linked it with an incomplete (and potentially misleading) concept of the 'laws of biology'. I will be specific.

On page 224 – under the heading of *Know Thyself* – he defines a soul in terms of it being 'the locus of *sentience, reason, and will* (assertion A). He avers that the soul consists of the information-processing activities of the brain (assertion B) and that this organ , i.e. the brain, is governed by 'the laws of biology' (assertion C).

The concept of an immaterial spirit is (i) an artifice that cannot be reconciled by the science of brain activity (assertion D) and (ii) the 'intuitive and morally useful' concept of an immaterial spirit cannot be reconciled with the 'scientific concept of brain activity' (assertion E).

There is one key phrase on this page which, in my opinion, opens the door to the dispelling of this welter of misconception and incompleteness: it is 'the laws of biology'. Who could dispute that the laws of biology are provided by physics and chemistry? The question is rhetorical because physics has been compelled to posit at least four levels of subatomic particles.

The neural networks are formed by the material neurons and their synapses, together with the fermions and bosons which subtend them. But quarks and leptons are part and parcel of foundations of the organizing layer which <u>subtends</u> that layer!

To me, the line of demarcation between the sets of levels runs close to Guy Lyon Playfair's 'Indefinite Boundary' – the two sets are separated by a distance measurable in terms of orders of magnitude, and scientists start talking of relational holism or holistic dualism/ dualistic holism, etc.

Ultimately, everything reduces to comparatively simple mathematics effecting a 'dualism of properties'. I refer to differences in spin, or sign, or polarity, and to such things as symmetry and supersymmetry. In short, the kind of subjects that so interest Roger Penrose.

In my opinion, therefore, an incalculable amount of thought, practice, and experience is sacrificed to produce an argument that is flimsy, untenable, and even deleterious to mankind.

Cormack, R.M. (1971), *The Statistical Argument*, Oliver and Boyd, Edinburgh.

Cox, David (1973), ANALYTICAL PSYCHOLOGY, Teach Yourself Books.

       The English Universities Press, London.

Crick, Joyce (1999), *SIGMUND FREUD: THE INTERPRETATION OF DREAMS*

       [A New Translation emphasizing words and semiotics],

       Oxford University Press.

Croxton *and* Cowden, (1963), *Applied General Statistics*. Pitman, London.

Daintith, J. & Rennie, R. (Eds.), (2005), *The Facts On File DICTIONARY of MATHEMATICS*, Facts on File, Inc., New York.

Daintith, John, Editor (2003), *The facts of file DICTIONARY of BIOCHEMISTRY*, Checkmark Books, New York.

Samasio, Antonio (2000), *The Feeling of What Happens…*, Heinemann.

       [This completes the set of neurophysiologists whose *all* favour MacKay's notion of the mechanization of mind-like processes, from Sherrington's 'ultimate pontifical nerve cell' to MacKay's 'Determinator', and again 'selves' and 'nonconscious neural patterns' can b cross-correlated with ideas in other disciplines]

Davies, Paul (1995), *ABOUT TIME*, Viking, PENGUIN, England.

--------   (1987), *SUPERFORCE*, Unwin Paperbacks, London.

--------Ed.   (1990), *The New Physics*, CUP.

Davies, P. and Hersh R., (1986), *DESCARTES' DREAM…*, Penguin, London.

Davies, P. & Gribbin, J.   (1991), *the matter myth…*, Viking.

Deikman, Arthur (1977), *Finding your way to the real world*, Souvenir Press.

Deutsch, D. (1997), *THE FABRIC OF REALITY,* Allen Lane, Penguin Press..

Devereux, George Editor (1953), *PSYCHOANALYSIS and the OCCULT*, Souvenir

       Press, London.

Eysenck, H.J. (1962), *Uses and Abuses of Psychology*, Pelican.

Field, M. and Golubitsky, M. (1992), *SYMMETRY IN CHAOS,* OUP.

FREUD AND JUNG

The encephalization of Mind brings the ideologies of Freud and of Jung close together, to such an extent that Jung's depiction of Personality amplifies Freud's depiction of the conscious Ego. Jung eschewed personal love and preferred to mention (briefly) cosmogonic love (which he assigned to God), whereas Freud _did_ care about personal love – for the Other.

For him, 'Eternal Eros' meant the love for others that finds its expression in the relations we form with those who are important to us and in what we do to make a better life, a better world for them. Bruno Bettelheim argues that, of all the mistranslations that have hampered our understanding of Freud's meaning, none has done more damage than the elimination of his references to the soul.

We see the stark contrast in this. For Jung, the goal of the psyche is the Self: for Freud, it is the Other. Freud, it seems, was much better suited to deal with matters pertaining to a world consisting only of relationships and fields. And yet – both were worried about Man's Soul. Bettelheim's book is entitled _Freud & Man's Soul_, and Jung, in _Memories, Dreams, Reflections_, is concerned about the loss of 'the transcendence of the Christian myth' (p. 303.

In fact, both men were concerned about much the same thing – evil as determinant reality – Freud was Other-centred, Jung was Self-centred. I was really making a point about myths, but they (and their misuse) do figure largely in the battle for Man's soul. And, I am obliged to point out Bettelheimer's book by my desire for Rigour and Comprehensiveness.

Other books on Freud and Jungian theory are by

Jung: Papadopoulos & Saayman (Eds.); Storr; Fordham; Cox

Freud: Stafford-Clark; Bettelheim

Edel, L. (1982), _STUFF OF SLEEP AND DREAMS_, Chatto and Windus, London.

Edwards, W. & Tversky, A. (1967), _DECISION MAKING_, Penguin Books.

Evans, Dylan (2001), _Emotion_, OUP.

Eysenck, H.J. (1958),_Sense and Nonsense in Psychology_, Pelican.

Fordham, Frieda (1970), _An Introduction to Jung's Psychology_, Pelican.

Ferris (Ed.), Timothy (1991), _The World Treasury of PHYSICS< ASTRONOMY,
            and MATHEMATICS_, Little, Brown and Company.

Fitzgerald, E. (c1860), _The Rubyatof Omar Khayyam_, Miscellaneous.

Freud, Sigmund (1952), *Introductory Lectures on Psychoanalysis*,

        Allen and Unwin, London.

---------   (1957), *New Introductory Lectures on Psychoanalysis*,

        Hogarth Press; Institute of Psychoanalysis

---------   (1959), *Outline of Psychoanalysis*,

        Hogarth Press; Institute of Psychoanalysis.

---------   (1974), *Two Short Accounts of Psycho-Analysis*, Pelican.

Fromm, Erich (1972), *Psychoanalysis and Religion*, Bantam.

Gay, Peter (1986), *FREUD FOR HISTORIANS*, OUP.

Gathercole, C.E. (1969), *Assessment in Clinical Psychology*, Penguin.

Gell-Mann, M. (1994), *The Quark and the Jaguar*, Little, Brown, & Co., UK.

George, F.H. (1976), *CYBERNETICS*, Teach Yourself Books/Hodder &

        Stoughton, GB.

Glassman, William E, (2002), Approaches to Psychology, Open University

        Press, Buckingham.

Goleman, Daniel (2006), *Social Intelligence*, Hutchinson/Random House.

        [also *Emotional Intelligence, etc.*]

Good, I. J. (1950), *Probability and The Weighing of Evidence*. London: Griffin.

Greene, Brian (2004), *The Fabric of the Cosmos*, Penguin/Allen Lane, GB.USA.

Gregory, (Ed.) R. (1987), *THE OXFORD COMPANION TO THE MIND*, OUP.

Gribbin, John (1995), *SCHRODINGER@S KITTENS...*, Weidenfeld & Nicolson.

-----------   (2009), *In Search of the MULTIVERSE*, Allen Lane/ Penguin.

Griffiths (Ed.), A. Phillips (1973), *KNOWLEDGE AND BELIEF*, OUP.

Hall, Calvin S. (1961), *A PRIMER OF FREUDIAN PSYCHOLOGY*, Mentor Books

        The World Publishing Company, New York.

Hamlyn, D.W. (1983), *Perception, Learning and the Self*, Routledge & Kegan

        Paul, London, et al.

Hare, R.M. (1982), *Plato*, Oxford University Press, Oxford.

Hardy, Alister (1975), *The Biology of God.* Jonathan Cape, London.

Harre, R. (1965), *An Introduction to the Logic of the Sciences*, Macmillan.

Harris, Thomas A. (1973), *I'M OK – YOU'RE OK*, Pan Books, London.

Harrison, K.W., Probability, Judgment and Mind, (Vols. 23-4, Series in *The Journal of Naval Science*).

...c1967, A Use for Plausibility in Radar Probability Theory, *JNS*, Vol. 21, No. 6

...c1967, Asymptotic Growth Curvesin the Assessment of Radar Performance, *JNS Vol. 22, No. 6*

...c1968, Further Applications of the Logistic Function, *JNS* Vol. 23, No. 6.

...Mar. 1968, The Power of the Logistic Function, *JNS* Vol. 23, No. 2.

... The Logistic Function as a Mathematical Function in Underwater Physiology *(ASWE /XRS/13.19/35/68)*

...Automation and Sex Differences in Situation Appraisal (ARE AXT Tm 87001, Jan 1987)

...User Models and the Psychology o Command: Part One – The Systems Background *ARE TM(AXT) 87011 July 1987*

...User Models and the Psychology of Command Part Three – A Dual Approach to User Analysis, *ARE TM(AXT) 87013, Sept. 1987*

...User Models and the Psychology of Command: Part Two – User Analysis and Model Construction *ARE TM(AXC) 87012, Nov. 1987*

Hawking, S. & Penrose, R. (1997), *THE NATURE OF SPACE AND TIME*, Princeton University Press, Chichester, England.

Hobson, Peter (2002), *The CRADLE of THOUGHT*, MACMILLAN.

Hodgson, D. (1991), *THE MIND MATTERS*, OUP, New York.

Hofstadter, D.

Hollingdale, R.J. (1972), *Arthur Schopenhauer ESSAYS AND APHORISMS*, Penguin Books.

Hollis, Martin (1973), *The Light of Reason*, Fontana (Collins), London.

Holroyd, Stuart (1977), *PSI AND THE CONSCIOUSNESS EPLOSION*, Bodley Head, London.

Horgan, John (2000), *THE UNDISCOVERED MIND*, Phoenix (Orion Books).

Humphrey, N. (1984*), CONSCIOUSNESS REGAINED,* OUP.

Hunter, Ian (1958), *Memory*, Pelican.

Hutin, Serge (1972), *Astrology*, Tom Stacey Ltd., London.

Huxley, Aldous (1981), *THE HUMAN SITUATION*, Triad (Granada).

Iverson, J. (1977), *MORE LIVES THAN ONE,* Pan Books Ltd., London.

Jackendoff, Ray (1985), *Semantics and Cognition*, The MIT Press.

James, William (1963), *The Varieties of Religious Experience*, Fontana,
                 (Collins).

Jahn (Ed.), Robert G. (1981), *The Role of Consciousness in the Physical World*,
                 Westview Press, Boulder, Colorado.

Johnston, W. (1976), *SILENT MUSIC*, Fontana (Collins), G.B.

-------------   (1981), *THE INNER EYE OF LOVE*, Fount Paperbacks, London.

Jung, C.G. (1964), *Memories, Dreams, Reflections*, Readers Union, Collins and
                 Routledge & (1972), Kegan Paul, London.

-------------(1972), *Four Archetypes*, Routledge & Kegan Paul, London.

Kaku, Michio (1994), *Hyperspace…*, Oxford University Press, Oxford.

Kalmus, H. (1954), *Genetics*, Pelican.

Kaufmann, Arnold (1968), *The Science of Decision-making…*, World
                 University Library, Weidenfeld and Nicolson, London.

Keehn, J.D. (1996), *MASTER BUILDERS OF MODERN PSYCHOLOGY*,
                 Duckworth, London.

Kennedy, Roger (2001), *Libido*, Icon Books, Cambridge.

King, Ursula (1980), *Towards a New Mysticism*, Collins, London.

Kosslyn, S.M. (1983), *Ghosts in the Mind's Machine*, Norton, NY.

Krauss, Lawrence, (1990) *The Fifth Essence,* Vintage, London.

Laing, R.D. (1973), *The Divided Self*, Pelican.

Langley, Russell (1968), *Practical Statistics*, Pan Books.

Lasch, C. (1985), *The Minimal Self...*, Pan.

Laszlo, Ervin (1993), *The Creative Cosmos*, Floris Books, Edinburgh.

Lederman, L. (1993), *THE GOD PARTICLE*. Bantam Press, Transworld
      Publishers Ltd.

Leff, Julian (2001), *THE UNBALANCED* MIND, Weidenfeld & Nicolson.

Leinfellner, W.

Le Shan, Lawrence (1980), CLAIRVOYANT REALITY, Turnstone Press.

Lewis, C. S. (1955), *THAT HIDEOUS STRENGTH*, Pan Books, Ltd., London.

------------- (1963), *THE FOUR LOVES,* Fonatana Books, Collins.

------------- ( ), *THE SCREWTAPE LETTERS, etc.*, Folio Society, London.

Livesey, P.J. (1986), *LEARNING AND EMOTION: A Biologiical Synthesis*,
      Lawrence Erlbaum Associates, London.

Lloyd, P; Mayes, A; et alia (1999), *Introduction to PSYCHOLOGY*,
      Diamond Books/ HarperCollins, London..

Lomas, Peter (2001), *The LIMITS of Interpretation*, Robinson, London.

Lorimer (Ed.), David (2001), *Thinking Beyod the Brain*, Floris Books.

Lovejoy,

Low, Anthony (1978), *LOVE'S ARCHITECTURE,* New York University
      Press (Gotham Library).

Ludwig, Emil (1973), *DOCTOR FREUD*, Manor Books, New York.

Lyndsay, D.

MacKay, D.

-------- (1967), *FREEDOM OF ACTION IN A MECHANISTIC UNIVERSE*, CUP.

--------(1980), *BRAINS< MACHINES & PERSONS*, Collins, London.

--------(1991), *BEHIND THE <u>EYE</u>*, Basil Blackwell, Ltd., UK and USA.

Marcuse, F.L. (1961), *HYPNOSIS...*, Pelican.

MATHEMATICS and STATISTICS

Cantor, G.   Structured Infinity and the Transfinite

Penrose   Attributes and Functions Underlying the Material Realm

             Mathematical Platonism

Rucker Structures and Functions of the Transfinite

Good   Subjective Probability and the Weighing of Evidence

Brownlee   Analysis of Variance and Examples of Bayse's Theorem

Davies (Ed) Design and Analysis of industrial Experiments

Hicks   Fundamental Concepts in the Design of Experiments

THE LOGISTIC FUNCTION

Von Bertalanffy – General Applicability as a Growth Function

Croxted and Cowden – Non-Linear Growth and 'Hiving-Off'

Harrison   - Transformation Leading to Subjective Probability

----

Mattessich, R. (1978), *INSTRUMENTAL REASONING AND SYSTEMS METHODOLOGY*, D. Reidel Publishing Co., Holland.

May, Rollo (1977), *LOVE & WILL,* Fountain Books, Collins.

McGinn, Colin (1982), *THE CHARACTER OF MIND*, OUP, Oxford.

McGuire; McGlashan (1979), *THE FREUD/JUNG LETTERS*, Picador (Pan).

McRae (Ed.) (1971), *Management information systems*, Penguin Books.

Miller (Ed.), David (1983), *A POCKET POPPER*, Fontana.

Miller (Ed.) Jonathan (1983), *States of Mind*, BBC, London.

Mons, W.E.R. (1983), *BEYOND MIND,* Rider & Co., London, Australia, NZ.

Motoyama, H.(1992), *KARMA AND REINCARNATION,* Judy Piatkus, London.

Munroe, Ruth, L. (1957), *SCHOOLS OF PSYCHOANALYTIC THOUGHT,*

HUTCHINSON MEDICAL PUBLICATIONS, London.

Murray, David J. (1983), *A History of Western Psychology*, Prentice-Hall, NJ.

MYSTICISM

Johnston, W.   The Roads of East and West; Neurological Basis

Mons, W. E. R.   Resting Content with TEILHARD; Jung

Motoyama, H. The Hindu Yogic Tradition; Parallels with Christianity

Ouspensky, P. D.   Intuitive Logic; Dimensional Time

Polkinghorne, J.   Christian-Orientated Science and Philosophy

Rucker, R.   The Infinite; the Transfinite; the One and the Many

------

Newell, R.W. (1986), *Objectivity, Empiricism and Truth*, Routledge &
          Kegan Paul, London.

Newman, James (1956), The World of MATHEMATICS, *Simon and Schuster*.

Oakley, D.A. Ed. (1985), *Brain & Mind*, Methuen, London.

O'Neill, T. (1980), *The Individuated Hobbit*, Thames & Hudson, London.

Ornstein (Ed.) R.E. (1973), *The Nature of Human Consciousness*,
          W.H. Freeman & Co., San Francisco, California.

Ornstein, R.E.   (1972), *THE PSYCHOLOGY OF CONSCIOUSNESS*,
          W.H. Freeman & Co., San Francisco, California.

Ouspensky, P.D. (1970), *TERTIUM ORGANUM*, Routledge & Kegan Paul,
          London.

Pagels, Heinz, R. (1983), *The Cosmic Code...*, Michal Joseph, London.

Papadopoulos K., and Saayman G, Eds. (1991), *JUNG IN MODERN
          PERSPECTIVE...*, PRISM PRESS, Bridport, Dorset.

Paton, H.J. (1981), *The Moral Law* [Kant], Hutchinson, London.

Peat, F. David (1988), *SUPERSTRINGS...*, Scribners (Macdonald), London.

Person, E.S. (1989), *LOVE and Fateful Encounters...*, Bloomsbury, London.

Peterson, Ivars (1990), *Islands of Truth...*, Freeman & Co., NY.

Pinker, Steven (2002), *THE BLANK SLATE*, Allen Lane/Penguin.

------------   (2007), *The STUFF of THOUGHT*, Allen Lane/Penguin.

        [Pinker excludes the pragmatics underlying Sino-Asiatic models and the enormous power of computer models.   His ignorance of real-time, computer-based, 'Command Support Systems' and their parallels with the brain is even greater than that of Ernest Kent – see 'Computer Systems' in this Bibliography]

Platts, M. (1979), *Ways of Meaning*, Routledge & Kegan Paul.

Playfair, G.L. (1977), *THE INDEFINITE BOUNDARY*, Panther, St. Albans, Herts.

Polkinghorne, J. (1984), *THE QUANTUM WORLD*, Longman Inc., New York.

....   (1988), *SCIENCE AND CREATION...*, SPCK, London.

Popper K. & and Eccles J. (1977), *The Self and Its Brain*, Springer-Verlag.

Preiss (Ed.), Byron (1989), *THE MICROVERSE*, Bantam Books, Byron Preiss VP.

Priestley, J. B. (1964), *Man & Time*, Aldus Books Ltd., Great Britain.

Radford, John & Govier, Ernest (1995), *A TEXTBOOK OF PSYCHOLOGY*,

        Routledge, London.

Ratey, John (2001), *A USER'S GUIDE TO THE BRAIN*, Little, Brown & Co.

Reed, T.J, (1984), *GOETHE*, OUP.

Reid, Constance (1963), *A LONG WAY FROM EUCLID*, Thom. Crowell Co. NY.

Ridley, Matt (2003), *nature via nurture*, Fourth Estate (HarperCollins).

Robinson, J. (1974), *But that I Can't Believe*, Fontana.

Robinson, Marilynne (2010), *Absence of Mind*, Yale University Press,

        [includes a lecture on the 'Freudian Self' and Jung]

Rose, S. (2005), *THE 21st-CENTURY BRAIN...*, Jonathan Cape.

        [mentions Delgado]

---------   1976), *THE CONSCIOUS BRAIN*, Pelican.

Rose, Kamin, and Lewontin, (1984), *NOT IN OUR GENES*, Pelican.

Rose, Sten (1997), *LIFELINES*, Allen Lane (Penguin).

[A materialistic argument compatible with mathematical

Platonism as it is in MacKay's Comprehensive Reality]

Rucker, R. (1982), *INFINITY & THE MIND*, Harvester Press, Brighton, Sussex.

.... (1986), *THE FOURTH DIMENSION...*, Penguin Books.

Russell, Bertrand (1983), *A HISTORY OF WESTERN PHILOSOPHY*, Allen &

Unwin.

Rycroft, Charles (1972), *A critical Dictionary of PSYCHOANALYSIS*,

Penguin Books.

------------ (1973), *anxiety and neurosis*, Pelican.

Ryle, Gilbert (1976), *THE CONCEPT OF MIND*, Peregrine Books (Penguin).

Savage, L.J. (1964), *Statistical Inference*, Methuen, London.

Sawyer, W.W. (1963), *Prelude to Mathematics*, Pelican/Penguin.

----------- (1954), *Mathematicians Delight*, Pelican.

Scientific American (1993), *MIND AND BRAIN*, W.H. Freeman, New York.

Seltman, C. (1956), *WOMEN IN ANTIQUITY*, Great Pan.

----------- (1952), *THE TWELVE OLYMPIANS...*, Pan.

Sheldrake, Rupert (2003), *THE SENSE OF BEING STARED AT*, Hutchinson,

London.

Singer, Peter (1989), *HEGEL*, OUP.

[Peter Singer explains how Hegel used the same word to describe
'mind' and 'spirit'. This, he says, leads to a reasonable case for *panentheism*. John
Polkinghorne makes the same case for a Christian viewpoint on this. Hegel's case is
consonant with Platonism]

Sloman, Aaron (1978), *THE COMPUTER REVOLUTION IN PHILOSOPHY...*,

Harvester Press, (John Spiers), Hassocks, Sussex.

Smolin, Lee (2000), *Three Roads to QUANTUM GRAVITY*, Weidenfeld and

Nicolson, London.

Solomon, Robert C. (1993), *THE PASSIONS: Emotions and the meaning of Life.*

Hackett Publishing Company, Indianapolis/Cambridge.

Spencer Brown, G. (1958), *Probability and Scientific Inference*, Longmans,

    Green, and Co., London.

Sprott, W.J.H. (1967), *Human Groups*, Penguin.

Stafford-Clark, David (1961), *PSYCHIATRY TODAY*, Pelican Books.

----------- (1967), *What Freud Really Said*, Pelican Books.

Steinbeck, J. (1979), *THE ACTS OF KING ARTHUR AND HIS NOBLE KNIGHTS*,

    Book Club, Associates.

Stevens, A. (1998), *AN INTELLIGENT PERSON'S GUIDE TO PSYCHOTHERAPY*,

    Gerald Duckworth, London.

Stewart, Ian (1995), *NATURE'S NUMBERS*, Basic Books (HarperCollins) NY.

Storr, Anthony (1973), *Jung*, Fontana/Collins.

Strawson (Ed.), P.F. (1973), *PHILOSOPHICAL LOGIC*, OUP.

Sturrock, John (1986), *STRUCTURALISM*, Paladin Grafton Books/Collins.

Sulloway, F.J, (1979), *FREUD, BIOLOGIST OF THE MIND...*, Fontana, GB.

Sutherland, Stuart (1992), *IRRATIONALITY The Enemy Within*, Constable & Co.

    London.

SUPERSYMMETRY

I have consulted mostly the works of three separate authors on this. They are, in no particular order, Roger Penrose, F.David Peat, and Jim Al-Khalili. Their opinions differ, but it suffices to address Roger Penrose's reference to Nature and to align the others to it.

In *The Road to Reality* (2004, p. 873), he is 'totally unconvinced' of the _physical_ (my emphases) relevance of predicted schemes of supersymmetry to what has been observed in Nature. And, from his previous works, this appears to be totally at odds with his views on neural nets, neurons, non-computability, etc. which are surely features of Nature.

Moreover, neurons, etc., can be reduced to differences between fermions and bosons, or, even deeper, between leptons and quarks. Or, more basically, differences of mathematical sign between particles. These levels are well attested as correlating strongly with 'natural' phenomena.

David Peat (285-6) points out the stability of the subatomic world makes us certain [his term] of the stability of compactified dimensions. Also, that supersymmetry links fermions and bosons together, thus affording us the possibility of 'further unification' involving 'supergravity' via gravity.

Jim Al-Khalili refers specifically to Nature in saying that 'we simply don't know yet whether nature behaves in a supersymmetric way'. It may be, he continues, that supersymmetry has a more fundamental role to play which would make grand unified theories seem *parochial in comparison*.

A fourth, very useful, reference that I must give is Michio Kaku's *Hyperspace*. This relates to the 'exciting possibilities' of *sparticles* which are the supersymmetric partners of ordinary partices. For example, the supersymmetrical partners of the quark and the leptron, respectively, are the *squark* and the *sleptron* (p. 145). Worthy of remark, also, are Kaku's words on gravity, spin, etc., (p. 144).

And, finally a quotation:-

'All that is needed to construct any material object, from the simplest atom to the most delicious wine, are *u*'s, *d*'s, and *e*'s: up quarks, down quarks, and electrons'

(Alvaro de Rujula, CERN)

SYMBOLOGY

It is clear that, by postulating a *psyche* that is non-material, Jung ruled out rigorous investigation of it as a system. Such an opinion is justified by the examination of Jung's recourse to the Sino-Asiatic concepts of the Mandala and the YIN and the YANG principles, echoed by his disciples, as it is shown in *Man and his Symbols*.

This, as recognized by Timothy O'Neill, is extremely important because it has already reached down into psychotherapeutic practice. And, it could have been corrected had it been perceived that the Mandala (in this Jungian context) applies to systems that are deeper (further along an axis of Scale) than the YIN and the YANG, which are released in the physical universe (see Motoyama).

Thus, here, I indicate two authorities on Symbolism whose words are very relevant today, even though they were written half-a-century ago. One is a consultant psychologist (with Freudian leanings), and the other is a renowned biologist; both express their views on *Systems*. The former expert witness is Ruth L. Munroe, writing specifically on Jung's SYMBOLOGY and the latter is Ludwig von Bertalanffy.

I can think of no words better to describe the appositeness of von Bertalanffy ot the thrust of my thesis than 'an interdisciplinary approach to psychology, including biology, psychiatry, sociology, linguistics, economics, the arts, and other fields, of which the key words are *symbolism* and *system*, and which describes man as an organism operating as an *active personality system*'. [a compilation of words from the dust-jacket of *ROBOTS, MEN AND MINDS]*

In almost perfect complementarity, Ruth Munroe describes how she was approached by the director of The Dryden Press, because of her reputation as a psychologist who, having had close contacts with psychoanalysis, nevertheless regarded its practice as a kind of *patchwork eclecticism*'. She devotes thirty-six pages to Jung, of which three (pp. 572-574) are about Jung's theoretical 'psychology of symbols'. [I suggest that Dr. Munroe's words are equally apposite]

SYSTEMS THEORY

There are two books on this subject that I have read extensively, namely *General System Theory*, by Ludvig von Bertalanffy and *Instrumental Reasoning and Systems Methodology*, by Richard Mattessich. Both books have been recommended university text-books and I have found the former to be of more value than the latter.

Mattessich's book claims to be an 'Epistemology of the Applied and Social Sciences', and therein lie some of its weaknesses, in my opinion. I have already criticized Mattessich over his coverage of Subjective Probability, and I will give an example of a lack of depth in his book. From the number of authors quoted by Mattessich, his *reading* may have been sufficient but the communication of his *understanding* to the reader is insufficient.

I will give a specific case. Within three pages (53-5), he goes - via *concrescence* – from a *speculation* that the universe (reality, nature, world, cosmos, etc.) is made up of either a single *basic substance* (event) [his italics] or of a limited number of basic substances, to the *conclusion* that the 'ultimate justification' of the system approach should be sought in *a general representation of, (1) the process and result of physical, biological and social concrescence, and (2) the hierarchy and the feedbacks ensuing from these concretion processes.*

As a distinguished mentor told me, when I was a very young scientist, it's all very well feeling sure about such things, but you <u>do</u> have to demonstrate them. Mattessich clearly has Whitehead in mind, but Whitehead's system of thought is a set of metaphysical assertions. His ideas are splendid for use as a kind of 'sounding board', but not as a basis for ontological assumptions underlying a systems methodology.

For a work professing to be an 'epistemology of the applied and social sciences', attessich's book is completely and strikingly devoid of input from psychology, psychiatry, scientific branches of religions, mysticism, Sino-Asiatic yogic tradition, and Platonism. I recommend Ruth Munroe, Donald MacKay, Hiroshi Motoyama, William Johnston, and John Polkinghorne to remedy the deficiencies.

In short, I I much prefer von Bertalanffy's starting points of _categorizations, sets of differential equations, classification of information types,_ and so on.

Talbot, M. (1991),*THE HOLOGRAPHIC UNIVERSE*, Grafton Books, London.

Taylor, Gordon Rattray (1979), *The Natural History of the Mind*, Secker & Warburg, London.

Thomson, Robert (1959), *The Psychology of Thinking*, Pelican.

Thorpe, W.H. (1978), *Purpose in a world of Chance*, OUP, Oxford. New York.

Vajda, S. (1961), *The Theory of Games and Linear Programming*, Methuen.

Vernon, P.E. (1976), *Personality Assessment A Critical Survey*, Methuen.

Warwick, Kevin (2002), *I, CYBORG*, Century (Random House), London.

Wilczek, Frank (2009), *The LIGHTNESS of BEING*, Allen Lane (Penguin).

[Uses 'Grid' for 'the primary world-stuff' (p. 74)]

Wilson, G. and Nias, D. (1977), *LOVE'S MYSTERIES*, Fontana/Collins.

Whitehead, A.N. (1985), *Science and the Modern World*, Free Association Books, London.

Whitton, Joel and Fisher, Joe (1986), *LIFE BETWEEN LIFE*, Grafton/Collins.

Wildiers, N.M. (1971), *An introduction to TEILHARD de Chardin*, Fontana.

Will, C.M. (1988), *WAS EINSTEIN RIGHT?*, OUP.

Williamson, S. and Pearse, I.,(1965) *Science, Synthesis & Sanity*, Collins Clear-Type Press, London and Glascow.

Wilson, Colin (1985), *AFTERLIFE*, Harrap, London.

Wilson, Ed. Stephen (2003), *THE BLOOMSBURY BOOK OF THE MIND*, Bloomsbury, London.

Winston, Robert (2003), *the human mind...*, Bantam Press (Transworld.

Woolger, Roger J. (1999), *Other Lives, Other Selves*, Thorsons/HarperCollins.

[Links with Buddhist and Hindu perspectives, but also with Stanislav Grof. Their practises and precepts are utterly alien to Particle Physics, to Systems Theory and to Scale as a dimension. I mention them (a) for completeness of cover and (b) because their methodology extends into therapy]

Wynn Reeves, Joan (1958), *Body and Mind in Western Thought*, Pelican.

Zaehner, R.C. (1972), *DRUGS, MYSTICISM AND MAKE-BELIEVE*. Collins.

Zohar, Danah (1990), *The Quantum Self*, Bloomsbury, London.

Zukav, G. (1986), *THE DANCING WU LI MASTERS*, Flamingo/Fontana/Collins.